# FEED YOUR F*itness*

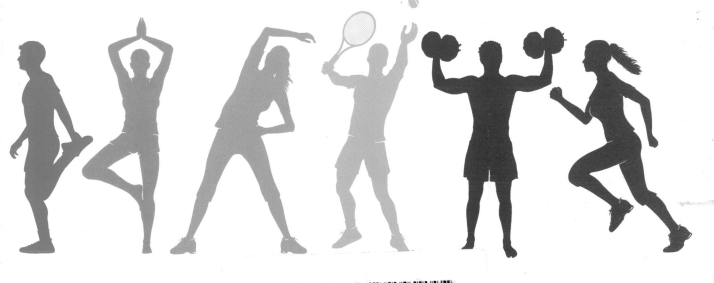

**DK** | Penguin
Random
House

**British Edition**
**Project Editors:** Caroline Curtis, Kathryn Meeker
**Senior Art Editor:** Glenda Fisher
**Angliciser:** Nikki Sims
**Editorial Assistant:** Amy Slack
**Design Assistant:** Rehan Abdul
**Pre-production Producer:** Rebecca Fallowfield
**Senior Producer:** Stephanie McConnell
**Creative Technical Support:** Sonia Charbonnier
**Managing Editor:** Stephanie Farrow
**Managing Art Editor:** Christine Keilty

**American Edition**
**Publisher:** Mike Sanders
**Associate Publisher:** Billy Fields
**Executive Acquisitions Editor:** Lori Cates Hand
**Production Editor:** Jan Lynn
**Cover and Book Design:** XAB Design
**Photographer:** Tom Hirschfeld
**Food Stylists/Chefs:** Tom Hirschfeld, Anthony Armstrong
**Indexer:** Johnna Dinse
**Layout:** Ayanna Lacey
**Proofreader:** Cate Schwenk

First Published in Great Britain in 2016 by
Dorling Kindersley Limited
80 Strand, London WC2R 0RL

Copyright © 2016 Dorling Kindersley Limited
A Penguin Random House Company
10 9 8 7 6 5 4 3 2 1
001–259430–Jan/2016

A CIP catalogue record for this book is available from the British Library.
ISBN: 978-0-2412-2976-7

Printed and bound in Slovakia.

All images © Dorling Kindersley Limited
For further information see: www.dkimages.com

A WORLD OF IDEAS:
**SEE ALL THERE IS TO KNOW**

www.dk.com

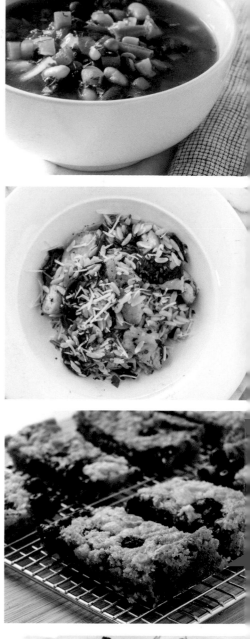

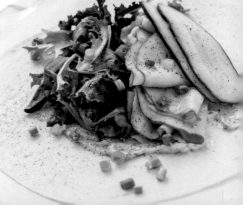

**ROWENA VISAGIE BSC** (MED) NUTRITION & DIETETICS, RD
**KARLIEN DUVENAGE** BSC DIETETICS, RD
**SHELLY MELTZER MSC** (MED) NUTRITION & DIETETICS, RD

# FEED YOUR *Fitness*

## A COOKBOOK TO FUEL HIGH PERFORMANCE

More than **80** easy-to-make, easy-to-eat, natural recipes for on-the-go athletes

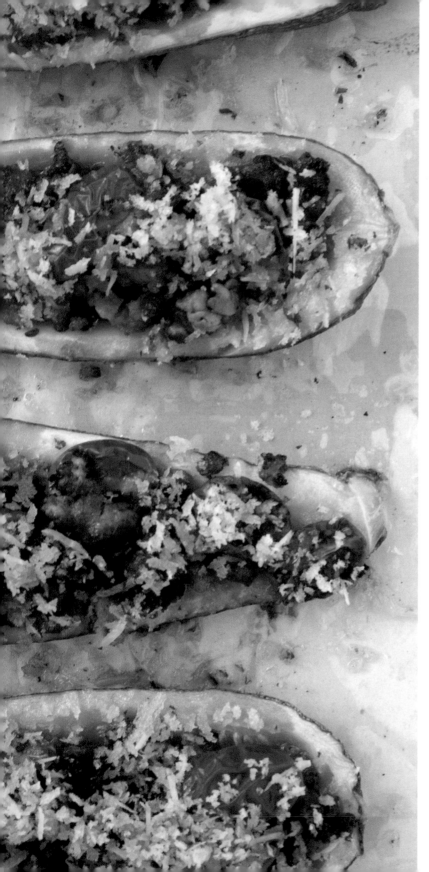

# Contents

**EGG AND AVOCADO
BREAKFAST BURRITOS**
Loaded with protein and
healthy fats for energy, satiety,
and cardiovascular health.

# Introduction

As an athlete, your body needs specific macro- and micronutrients to be a well-fuelled, powerful, athletic machine. But how do you get all those nutrients in your diet, and when should you consume them in relation to your workout or athletic event? How many calories do you need, and how do you break down all this information into specific meals?

We designed *Feed Your Fitness* to be your one-stop nutrition manual and cookbook for the athlete in you and in your family. In these pages, you have access to a wealth of nutritional knowledge as well as more than 80 power-packed recipes and variations to fuel your body.

You can learn the basics of nutrition, and why macronutrients (carbohydrates, proteins, and fats) as well as various micronutrients (vitamins and minerals) are important for every athlete. You can also explore fluids and electrolytes and the role they play in your performance on the field, in the gym, and more.

*Feed Your Fitness* provides specific information on the nutritional needs of both endurance and strength athletes and helps you choose the best foods for the type of sports you and your family members participate in. We help you stock your pantry, select essential cooking tools, and even give you hints on quick-cooking methods and meal assembly. We also provide easy-to-follow information on making real-food portables and homemade sports drinks and smoothies, leaving out all the mystery ingredients from shop-bought options.

A nutritional analysis is included for each recipe so that you can use them to help meet your dietary needs.

**ICONS**
The recipes in this book feature icons that point out recipes geared for specific nutritional needs:

**FAT CONSCIOUS**
Keeps calories down (fat is very calorie dense) to help prevent weight gain

**PROTEIN RICH**
Important for strength and rebuilding muscle

**CARBOHYDRATE RICH**
Provides important fuel for endurance and high intensity activities

**HIGH FIBRE**
Is ideal for larger meals 3–5 hours before activity

**EASILY DIGESTIBLE**
Best for digestion before and during training sessions and competitions

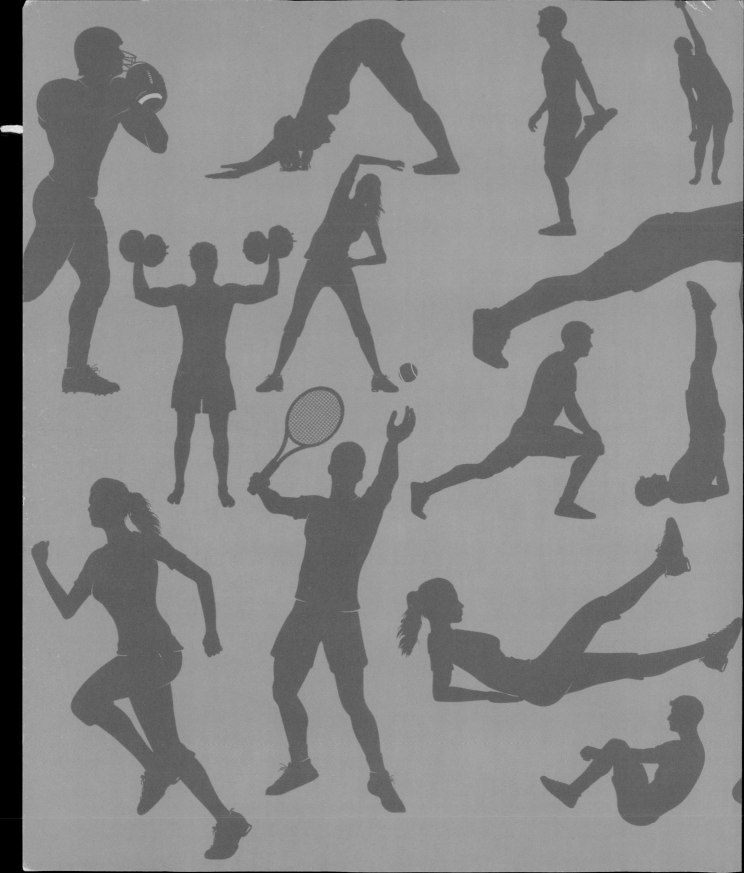

# Food for **Fitness**

Whether you're training for a sporting event like a triathlon or just working out at the gym, you need the right kind of fuel, in the right amount, at the right times. In the following pages we explain what you need to know in order to feed yourself the essential nutrients you need, when you need them.

To make the "feeding" part easier, we help you stock your kitchen with essential ingredients, and give you the tools you need to easily and efficiently prepare recipes. Finally, we give you quick-cooking and meal-assembly tips and pointers on preparing your own portables and sports drinks. Eating well has never been easier.

# From Food **to Fuel**

When you eat food, it goes through a series of chemical reactions inside your body, with the end products being carbon dioxide, water, heat, and energy in the form of a chemical called adenosine triphosphate (ATP). The energy needed to perform physical activity is produced from the breakdown of chemical bonds found in carbohydrates, proteins, and fats, and the production of ATP.

## WHERE ENERGY COMES FROM

Most energy is provided from the breakdown of carbohydrates and fats. Protein is rarely used as an energy source because the amino acids in protein are used for building and maintaining muscle, although the body can use protein as an energy source when carbohydrate intake is inadequate. The liver and muscles can store glucose as glycogen for later use as well as fat, in the form of intramuscular triglycerides, as an additional energy source.

Muscle cells also contain a chemical called phosphocreatine, which provides energy during high-power, short-duration activities that last a few seconds, such as sprinting, weightlifting, throwing, or a tennis serve. Muscle cells store only a small amount of phosphocreatine but can replenish ATP very quickly by donating phosphorus molecules to form new ATP molecules. Although this does not generate a large amount of ATP, it serves as an additional energy system to supply small amounts of ATP very quickly to muscle cells when the demand for energy is very high.

## THE PROCESS OF GLYCOLYSIS

As ATP is consumed, the by-products of this reaction begin to build up and trigger another energy system, glycolysis, to increase its ATP production. Glycolysis is an energy system that can only use glucose or glycogen for energy production. It can occur with or without the presence of oxygen.

Without adequate oxygen present, glycolysis typically lasts for 1–3 minutes. If intense physical activity continues, hydrogen ions (a by-product of glycolysis) start to accumulate and contribute to the formation of a molecule called lactate. Lactate is metabolized by skeletal and heart muscle to provide energy.

## MUSCLE SORENESS

Post-exercise muscle soreness is often blamed on high levels of lactate or lactic acid. However, this is not the case, and we now know that the real cause is an accumulation of hydrogen ions, causing a decrease in the body's pH, and a rise in muscle acidity. In fact, lactate is an important source of fuel – produced and used by the muscles, particularly during exercise.

## HOW ATP TRANSLATES TO PERFORMANCE

With adequate oxygen present, glycolysis produces ATP. Complete metabolism of 1 glucose molecule can produce 38 ATP molecules, which is equivalent to about 266 kilocalories (kcals) of available energy, or enough energy for a person weighing 81.5kg (180lb) to run at 4 miles per hour (6km/hour) for 30 minutes.

**FOOD TO ENERGY**
Through the process of digestion and absorption, macronutrients and micronutrients in food are broken down to be used by your body.

**MOUTH/SALIVARY GLANDS**
Saliva plus chewing breaks down food; carb and fat digestion begins here.

**OESOPHAGUS**
Transports food from the mouth to the stomach.

**LIVER**
Breaks down and synthesizes biological molecules; stores glycogen, vitamins, and iron; produces bile to help emulsify fats during digestion.

**GALLBLADDER**
Stores and concentrates bile.

**PANCREAS**
Secretes hormones to help regulate blood glucose levels; stores and secretes enzymes to aid digestion of proteins, carbs, and fats.

**STOMACH**
Stores food and continues digestion with the help of enzymes and hydrochloric acid; helps kill bad bacteria.

**LARGE INTESTINE**
Completes absorption of vitamins, minerals, and water, and conducts bacterial fermentation and faeces formation.

**SMALL INTESTINE**
Completes digestive process and conducts absorption of carbs, protein, fats, vitamins, and minerals.

**RECTUM**
Stores and expels faecal material.

**ANUS**
Opening for eliminating faecal material.

# Determining Your **Energy Requirements**

Proper nutrition is essential for maximizing performance and to meet the energy demands of training and competition. Inadequate nutrition can limit training gains, which impairs performance and overall health. The following are some important topics to consider when determining nutritional needs.

## BASAL ENERGY EXPENDITURE

Basal energy expenditure (also known as BEE) is the amount of energy your body uses to carry out fundamental metabolic functions, such as breathing, kidney function, and blood circulation, in a resting state. Genetics, age, gender, weight, lean body mass, and fat mass all can affect basal energy expenditure.

Women typically have more body fat and less muscle mass than men. Because fat is less metabolically active than muscle, this results in a lower basal energy expenditure for women.

Basal energy expenditure makes up 60–75 per cent of daily energy needs and typically declines as you age due to a loss of muscle mass. Another 10 per cent of daily energy is spent on digesting and metabolizing food, which is called the thermic effect of food.

## ENERGY BALANCE

Consuming more calories than your total daily energy expenditure results in weight gain, typically in the form of fat. About 0.5kg (1lb) of fat is equivalent to 14,700kJ (3,500kcal). Eating fewer calories and exercising or burning more calories can result in safe weight loss. Consuming 2,000 fewer kilojoules (500kcal) a day equals 14,700kJ (3,500kcal) a week, enough to lose 0.5kg (1lb) of fat. Burn an additional 2,000kJ (500kcal) a day through exercise, and you could lose 1kg (2lb) a week safely. As a general rule, it is not advised to lose more than 0.5–1kg (1.1–2.2lb) a week.

## ENERGY AVAILABILITY CONCERN

When athletes restrict energy in order to lose body fat, they should do so gradually. Severe restriction of energy intake can lead to metabolic, reproductive, and bone disorders. This is usually a result of a low energy availability. Energy availability is the amount

**GREEN SALAD**
Eating plenty of vegetables is a low-calorie way to get important nutrients.

**DAILY ENERGY EXPENDITURE** (kJ/kcal burned per day)

The following chart shows how your total amount of energy is spent in a typical day. Physical activity is the area you have the most control over and can manipulate.

**THERMIC EFFECT OF FOOD**
(digestion, absorption, and metabolism of food): **10%**

**BASAL ENERGY EXPENDITURE**
(breathing, circulation, kidney function, etc.): **60–70%**

**PHYSICAL ACTIVITY: 20–30%**

of energy available for body functions (e.g. growth and reproduction), after the energy used during exercise is subtracted from the energy obtained from your diet. A low energy availability means you do not have enough energy for both body and exercise functions. This can also be caused by expending large amounts of energy in training and failing to compensate with an increased energy intake. To protect reproductive and bone health, energy availability should not fall below 125kJ (30kcal) per kilogram fat-free mass per day.

## BODY COMPOSITION

Body composition reflects the body fat and muscle mass that combine to make up your weight. Overall body composition can affect physical activity and athletic performance. Carrying excess body fat requires more energy to move the excess weight. Expending these extra calories can decrease aerobic or endurance athletic performance. Unlike muscle, excess fat does not produce force. So, having more fat results in less force production, but requires more energy, as you have more weight to move. This can decrease overall speed of movement. However, an "ideal" body composition may differ for different sports (e.g. extra body fat can help open-water, long-distance swimmers by providing extra buoyancy and warmth; and different positions in rugby require varying amounts of body fat for protection).

## PREFERRED TOOLS TO ASSESS BODY COMPOSITION IN ATHLETES

Generally, a measurement of body fat, using skinfold measurements, is all that is required when assessing an athlete's physique. Girths can be useful to measure body composition changes at the beginning and end of a strength training or weight loss programme. The body mass index (BMI) does not differentiate between lean body mass and body fat, so is not sensitive to changes in body composition, and therefore should not be used for monitoring athletes.

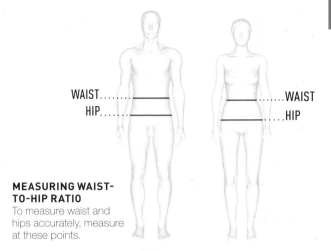

**MEASURING WAIST-TO-HIP RATIO**
To measure waist and hips accurately, measure at these points.

## CALCULATING YOUR ENERGY NEEDS

Several mathematic equations are used to estimate kilojoule or calorie needs, and you can find calculators online. The following table offers easy equations to determine your kilojoule needs using the kilojoule-per-kilogram* method. However, for best results, it is recommended that athletes seek individual advice from a dietitian or nutritionist with sports experience.

| Goal | Equation |
|------|----------|
| Weight loss | Weight in kg × 104kJ (25kcal) |
| Weight maintenance | Weight in kg × 125kJ (30kcal) |
| Weight gain | Weight in kg × 146kJ (35kcal) |

*1kg is equal to 2¼lb. So, to determine your weight in kg, divide your weight in pounds by 2.25.*

## BODY FAT PERCENTAGES

The following body fat ranges should be seen as a guide only, as they do not account for individual genetic variability or specific sports and playing positions. It is also important to remember that body composition is only one factor contributing to performance.

| | Men | Women |
|------|------|-------|
| Essential fat | 5% | 12% |
| Athletes | 5–14% | 12–23% |
| Acceptable | 15–20% | 24–30% |
| Overweight | 21–24% | 31–36% |
| Obese | 25% or greater | 37% or greater |

# Nutrition **Basics**

Nutrition plays a fundamental role in sport – to supply fuel for energy, as well as all the essential nutrients and fluid. In this section we look at the different macronutrients (carbohydrate, protein and fat) and the micronutrients (vitamins and minerals), as well as fluid and electrolytes, and their roles in sports performance.

## CARBOHYDRATES

Consisting of sugars, starches, and fibre, carbohydrates (or carbs) are found in fruits, dairy, grains, starchy vegetables (such as potatoes, sweet potatoes, corn, and peas), and legumes.

Carbohydrate digestion begins in the mouth and takes place primarily in the small intestine. Broken-down carbohydrates are absorbed in the small intestine and transported to the liver, where glucose is stored as glycogen. When extra energy is needed, the liver can break down the stored glycogen to maintain normal blood glucose levels. Glucose may be used immediately for energy for a workout, or it can be stored as glycogen or fat.

For most athletes, carbohydrates are the body's preferred fuel source, especially as the intensity of their activity increases.

## PROTEIN

Good sources of protein include lean beef, pork, chicken, turkey, fish, seafood, eggs, nuts, and nut butters. Many carbohydrate-rich foods like legumes and dairy products also contain protein.

Protein digestion takes place in the stomach and small intestine. Protein is eventually broken down into smaller amino acid molecules, which are absorbed in the small intestine and transported in the bloodstream. Once proteins are broken down into amino acids, they are used in the body as building blocks for the synthesis of hormones, enzymes, neurotransmitters, DNA (deoxyribonucleic acid), RNA (ribonucleic acid), and the structural components of muscle. Your body can synthesize some amino acids on its own, but there are some that your body must obtain through food.

### CLASSIFICATION OF CARBOHYDRATES ACCORDING TO THEIR USE IN SPORTS SITUATIONS

Carbohydrate quality varies according to the food source. This will also determine their use in sport. For an athlete, carbohydrates can be divided into the following categories:

| Types of carbohydrate | Examples | Use |
| --- | --- | --- |
| Nutrient-dense: these are also rich in other nutrients including vitamins and minerals, and some options provide protein, fibre, and antioxidants | Grains such as oats, quinoa, brown rice, couscous, cereals, and breads (it is best to choose wholegrains or high fibre most of the time); legumes; starchy vegetables ( such as potatoes, sweet potatoes, and corn); and dairy products | These should be chosen as part of an athlete's every day diet.<br><br>Lower fibre options may be better before and during exercise for gastrointestinal comfort. |
| Concentrated, fast-releasing: these are usually low in other nutrients | Sports drinks, gels, cordials, and sports sweets | Use should be limited to training sessions and competitions and/or when additional carbohydrates are needed (to counter low appetite or for weight gain). |
| High fat: foods that contain carbohydrate but are high in fat | Cakes, pastries, pies, crisps, fried chips, full cream milkshakes, ice-cream, and chocolate | Eat these as occasional treat foods. |

Protein provides the building blocks needed both to build and to repair muscle, which improves strength and power.

## FATS

Fats are found in all kinds of foods, such as oils, margarine, butter, nuts and nut butters, some fruits (avocados), dairy products (except those that are fat-free), beef, pork, poultry, and fish (particularly oily fish like salmon). Many processed foods are also rich sources of fat – e.g. cakes, pastries, pies, crisps, biscuits, sauces, fried foods, and crumbed foods.

Dietary fat is composed of different fatty acids – saturated, unsaturated (mono- and polyunsaturated) and trans fatty acids. Most fats contain a mixture of saturated and unsaturated fats. Different foods have varying proportions of fatty acids – meat, dairy and coconut contain predominantly saturated fat; olive and rapeseed oils, and avocado pears have a high proportion of monounsaturated fats; and sunflower and soya oils mostly consist of polyunsaturated fats. Essential fatty acids (omega-3 and 6) are a subgroup of polyunsaturated fats. Not all fats are equal – some are healthier than others. Trans fats, found in many processed foods and hard brick margarines, have been found to be harmful to our health, and are best avoided; whereas monounsaturated and omega-3 fatty acids (mostly found in oily fish) are particularly protective of heart health so their inclusion in the diet is preferential.

Fat digestion takes place primarily in the stomach and small intestine. Fatty acids are absorbed in the small intestine, incorporated into lipoproteins and

**FISH**
Fish is a good alternative source of protein to red meat.

**NUTS**
Walnuts are rich in omega-3 fatty acids, which help to promote heart and brain health.

chylomicrons, and then transported in the bloodstream. Lipoproteins contain fats bound to proteins, which help the compound move both through the bloodstream and in and out of cells more easily. Chylomicrons are part of a group of five lipoproteins (chylomicrons, very-low-density lipoprotein/VLDL, intermediate-density lipoprotein/IDL, low-density lipoprotein/LDL, and high-density lipoprotein/HDL) that contain triglycerides, phospholipids, cholesterol, and protein. These lipoproteins are used to transport dietary fats and cholesterol from the intestines to other areas in the body by way of the bloodstream.

Fatty acids not immediately used for energy production are stored as triglycerides in fat cells or inside muscle cells as intramuscular triglycerides. Through a process called lipolysis, the stored triglycerides are broken down into glycerol and three fatty-acid molecules and metabolized for energy.

Fats are a particularly important energy source for endurance athletes to preserve already-limited glycogen stores until they're needed while delaying fatigue and increasing exercise duration.

## VITAMINS AND MINERALS

These so-called micronutrients do not directly provide energy but are necessary for the body to conduct a number of metabolic processes, such as adequate growth and development, transport of oxygen, and proper immune function.

Certain vitamins and minerals also serve as antioxidants (e.g. vitamins A, C, and E and selenium), helping prevent free-radical damage in the body. Thiamin, riboflavin, niacin, vitamin $B_6$, folic acid, vitamin $B_{12}$, vitamin C, magnesium, zinc, copper, and iron are just some of the micronutrients that play key roles in a number of energy pathways in the body.

Being deficient in one or several vitamins or minerals could affect your body's ability to produce energy, impair your athletic performance, and compromise your health. Most athletes' diets have been shown to provide adequate vitamins and minerals, as long as they are varied and meet the athlete's energy needs. Situations which may increase risk include:

- prolonged, exhaustive exercise
- lengthy periods of restrictive energy intake
- exclusion of certain food groups (e.g. dairy, meat)
- training at altitude and extreme environmental conditions
- high losses through sweat, urine, and faeces.

Note: there is no evidence that supplementing a diet already sufficient in vitamins and minerals will improve performance or health. In fact, overdosing on micronutrients can be extremely harmful.

**CITRUS FRUITS**
Great sources of vitamin C, citrus fruits, such as tangerines, are also an easily portable snack.

## FLUIDS AND ELECTROLYTES

Maintaining adequate fluid and electrolyte intake during physical activity plays a significant role in optimizing performance. Excessive dehydration can increase the risk of bodily overheating, strain on the heart, increased perceived effort, loss of concentration, and gastrointestinal upset. However, overhydration can result in hyponatremia (low blood sodium levels caused by overdrinking), which can have serious health consequences like coma, seizures, and even death.

During exercise your muscles use 25 per cent of energy for work, while the remainder is released as heat (which is why we get hot during exercise). Our bodies increase the blood flow to our skin so the heat can be released via evaporation – sweating. The more you sweat, the more fluid you lose. There is also a loss of electrolytes, specifically sodium and chloride. Some people sweat more than others, which is why fluid requirements vary from person to person. Furthermore, the type of exercise, the exercise duration and intensity, fitness levels, gender, body size and composition, environmental conditions, and clothing can affect an individual's fluid needs.

Commercial sports drinks typically contain varying amounts of carbohydrate (some also contain protein and other ingredients like herbals and caffeine) and limited amounts of electrolytes (too much can affect the taste and so you may prefer foods with a high salt content, such as salted potatoes or pretzels). Specific fluid choice will depend on the type, intensity, and duration of your exercise as well as practicality, preference, and tolerance of solid foods versus fluid.

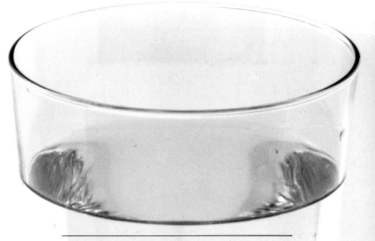

## TIPS FOR FLUID INTAKE

- Follow an individualized approach.
- Limit excessive body mass loss during exercise (you can monitor this during training by weighing yourself before and after sessions). Also, ensure there is no increase in body mass (this can indicate overhydration).
- Avoid overhydration by being sensitive to the onset of thirst as the signal to drink.
- Make the most of all opportunities to drink during exercise as needed.
- Have cool, palatable drinks that are easily accessible during training sessions. Each athlete should have their own personalized drinking bottle.
- Consider environmental conditions – the hotter it is, the more fluid you will need.

# Nutrition around **Training and Competition**

Training and competing seriously challenges your body's fuel stores, and the longer and/or the higher the intensity, the more your fuel stores are depleted. For this reason, fuelling correctly before, during, and after exercise is vital for optimal performance.

## CARBOHYDRATE

Carbohydrate is one of the main fuel sources used during exercise. You should aim to achieve carbohydrate intakes that will match the fuel needs of your training programme. You will also need to adequately replace your stores during recovery, between training sessions, and competitions.

## CARBOHYDRATE IN DAILY TRAINING DIET

Most athletes need to consume a diet high in carbohydrate to help replenish the muscles' glycogen stores. Your total carbohydrate intake depends on your training programme, body weight, and body composition goals, as outlined in the box opposite.

| DAILY TRAINING DIET | |
| --- | --- |
| **Situation** | **Daily carbohydrate needs** |
| Light training or need to reduce energy intake to lose weight | 3–5g per kg body weight |
| Moderate duration/ low-intensity training | 5–7g per kg body weight |
| Moderate to heavy endurance training | 6–10g per kg body weight |
| Extreme exercise programme (4–6+ hours per day) | 10–12g per kg body weight |

## CARBOHYDRATE INTAKE BEFORE ACTIVITY

Carbohydrate intake in the hours before a training session or competition will help to top up your liver's glycogen stores to ensure optimal fuel for performance.

The following guidelines for carbohydrate intake before activity are based on body weight and the amount of time before the exercise. These are just general guidelines, and gastric comfort should be taken into account as well. It is best to choose easily digestible foods before exercise to prevent any gastrointestinal issues. Always practice these strategies in training first.

To improve your performance, you should consume some carbohydrate during any physical activity that lasts 1 hour or longer. Carbohydrate intake during activity may provide an immediate fuel source, sparing the stored supplies of liver and muscle glycogen. For activity lasting 1–3 hours, it is recommended that you consume 30–60g of carbohydrate per hour.

Focus on easily digestible, fat conscious, and carbohydrate rich foods. Look for the recipes with these icons.

 **EASILY DIGESTIBLE**

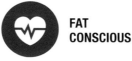 **FAT CONSCIOUS**

 **CARBOHYDRATE RICH**

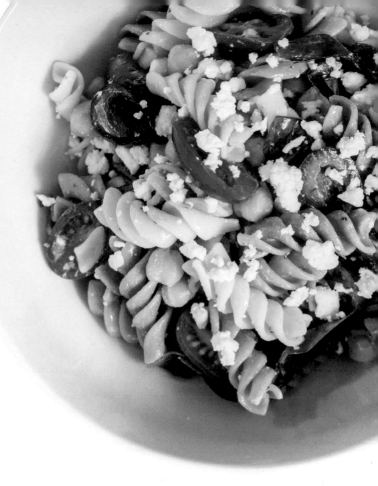

**GREEK PASTA SALAD**
This salad offers 46g of carbohydrate, 15g of protein, and 10g of fat.

During exercise lasting more than 3 hours, it has been found that up to 90g of carbohydrate can be tolerated, provided the carbohydrate is in different forms, known as multiple transportable carbohydrates (e.g. glucose + fructose). Small amounts of carbohydrate or even mouth rinsing with carbohydrate can improve performance during exercise lasting up to 1 hour.

## EXAMPLES OF PRE-EXERCISE MEALS AND SNACKS FOR AN 80KG (176LB) ATHLETE:

Use the following as a guide. Always experiment during training to find what works best for you and suits your gut.

### CARBOHYDRATE INTAKE BEFORE ACTIVITY

| Timing | Recommended carbohydrate intake | Example meal/snack |
|---|---|---|
| 3-4 hours before | 240-320g (3-4g/kg) | Large bowl oats porridge with low-fat milk, 1 banana and sugar/honey + 2 slices toast with jam + large glass fruit juice |
| 1-2 hours before | 80-160g (1-2g/kg) | 1 cereal bar + 1 fruit + 500ml sports drink |

Note: you will also need to consider gastric comfort.

### CARBOHYDRATE INTAKE BEFORE ACTIVITY

| Hours before exercise | Recommended carbohydrate intake |
|---|---|
| 1 | 1g per kg body weight |
| 2 | 2g per kg body weight |
| 3 | 3g per kg body weight |
| 4 | 4g per kg body weight |

| CARBOHYDRATES NEEDED DURING EXERCISE | |
|---|---|
| Length of event or training session | Recommended carboydrate intake |
| 30-60 mins | Mouth rinse |
| 1-3 hours | 30-60g per hour |
| >3 hours | Up to 90g per hour (must be multiple transportable carbohydrates e.g. glucose + fructose) |

## CARBOHYDRATE AFTER ACTIVITY

Carbohydrate is needed during the recovery phase - within 30–40 minutes of finishing exercise. During this phase, the enzyme that stimulates glycogen synthesis is elevated along with increased insulin sensitivity, both of which help promote rebuilding of glycogen stores. This is particularly important if there is less than 8 hours before the next training session or race.

Below are recommendations for carbohydrate intake after exercise. (Adding some protein may also help stimulate muscle protein synthesis, and if carbohydrate intake is insufficient, muscle glycogen restoration as well).

| CARBOHYDRATE INTAKE AFTER EXERCISE | |
|---|---|
| Consume carbohydrates within 30–40 minutes immediately after exercise to aid recovery, and eat more carbohydrates at regular intervals after this. | |
| Timing | Recommended carbohydrate intake |
| Immediately afterwards | 1.5g per kg body weight |
| 1 hour later | Additional 1.5g per kg body weight |

## CARBOHYDRATE LOADING

Carbohydrate loading is a strategy that can improve endurance performance by 20 per cent for some athletes when racing at high intensity for more than 90 minutes, by maximizing muscle glycogen stores and postponing fatigue. Latest protocols for carbohydrate loading involve increasing carbohydrate intake to 7–12g/kg body weight per day in the 24–36 hours prior to the event, and combining this with tapering and rest. If your appetite or gut tolerance limits your intake, wholegrains can be replaced with lower fibre (easily digestible) foods (such as plain cereals and tinned and peeled fruit), and high carbohydrate fluids (such as fruit juice, sports drinks, and smoothies) can be added. You may gain up to 2kg (4.5lb) whilst carbohydrate loading.

It may not even be necessary for some athletes to increase their carbohydrate intake if they consume sufficient carbohydrate in their usual diet. Instead, taper and rest may be adequate to maximize their glycogen stores.

It is important that an athlete practices their carbohydrate loading regimen well before important competitions.

## TRAIN LOW, COMPETE HIGH

This strategy has recently received some attention and is based on the theory that training with low carbohydrate stores or availability may enhance adaptations and increase the use of fat as a fuel. When carbohydrate stores are increased again before competition this may promote performance. "Training low" strategies can be achieved by training after an overnight fast, taking in less carbohydrate than required by your training session, drinking only water during a prolonged session, or not ingesting carbohydrate during recovery.

More research is needed to support that this strategy results in definite performance enhancement. There is also evidence that training low can result in an inability to train at high intensities. However, it may be a useful strategy for certain athletes, at certain training sessions, in particular phases of training (e.g. low-intensity sessions at the beginning of the training season).

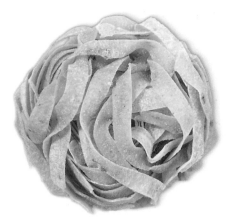

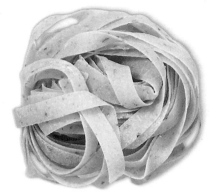

**TAGLIATELLE**
Pasta is a well-known source of carbohydrate and a traditional carbohydrate-loading choice for athletes.

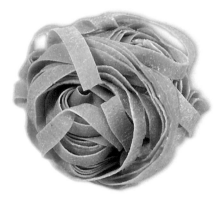

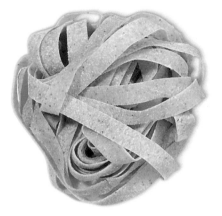

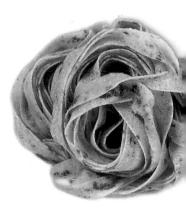

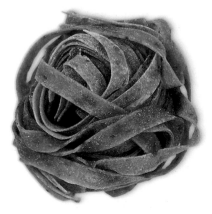

### WHAT ABOUT THE GLYCAEMIC INDEX?
The glycaemic index (GI) rates carbohydrate-rich foods according to how they raise blood glucose levels. High GI foods (e.g. white bread) raise blood glucose levels more quickly than lower GI foods (e.g. rye bread). Several factors affect the GI of a food, such as ripeness of the food, and how it was cooked or processed. The GI of a food is different when eaten alone, or in combination with other foods – adding fat or protein to a high GI food will lower the GI. Generally, in order to sustain energy levels and keep fuller for longer, you should include low GI foods in most meals; but during and immediately post training when you are wanting a quick source of fuel or rapid recovery of muscle glycogen stores, you may benefit from higher GI foods and drinks. However, use of the GI needs to be balanced with other nutritional principles such as portion size (total energy intake and specific amounts of carbohydrate, fat, and protein) and other important components of food such as fibre, vitamins, and minerals.

## THE POWER OF PROTEIN

Protein plays an important role in the response to exercise – particularly in the building of new tissue (including muscle) and repairing damaged tissue. If you are an endurance athlete involved in strenuous training, you will need extra protein to cover a small amount of the energy costs of your training and to enhance the recovery and muscle repair process after exercise. As a strength training athlete who would like to gain muscle, you will need more protein in the early stages of intensive resistance training. However, your muscles will adapt to the training and your requirements will only be a little higher than those that are generally active. If you are still growing (e.g. an adolescent), your protein requirements will be higher, and if you are female, your protein requirements may be 10–20 per cent lower than those for males.

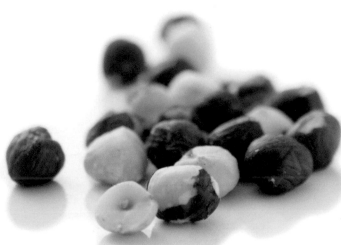

**HAZELNUTS**
Nuts are a convenient and portable source of protein to take along to endurance events.

| DAILY PROTEIN INTAKE RECOMMENDATIONS | |
|---|---|
| International sports medicine associations recommend the following protein intakes: | |
| **Group** | **Protein intake (g/kg body weight/day)** |
| Sedentary men and women | 0.8-1.0 |
| Recreational exercise | 0.8-1.0 |
| Moderate-intensity endurance training | 1.0-1.5 |
| Intensive endurance training | 1.5-2.0 |
| Power sports | 1.4-1.7 |
| Resistance training | 1.0-1.7 |
| Female Athletes | 10-20% less than males |

Look for recipes in this book with this icon, which signals a good source of protein.

 **PROTEIN RICH**

## PROTEIN INTAKE BEFORE AND DURING ACTIVITY

Evidence supporting the performance benefit of protein before and during exercise is inconclusive. However, consumption of protein post exercise has been shown to be of benefit, depending on recovery needs and goals.

## PROTEIN INTAKE AFTER EXERCISE

Consuming some protein together with carbohydrate in the recovery period promotes muscle synthesis and repairs muscle damage. An intake of protein immediately after exercise will enhance muscle uptake and retention of amino acids. This enhanced state of protein metabolism lasts for up to 24 hours; therefore, it is important for you to spread your protein intake throughout the rest of the day, as well as immediately after exercise. It is recommended that athletes ingest, on average, 20g of protein together with carbohydrate within 30 minutes after exercise for beneficial effects.

## FAT INTAKE RECOMMENDATIONS

Fats provide an additional source of energy for athletes. However, an overconsumption of calories from fat, particularly trans and some saturated fats, may increase the risk of chronic diseases. Experts recommend that you should limit your fat intake to between 20 and 35 per cent of your total calorie intake, and that saturated fat intake should only make up 10 per cent of total calories. However, make sure you consume no less than 20 per cent of fat to ensure an adequate intake of fat-soluble vitamins and essential fatty acids.

## ALCOHOL IN SPORT

Alcohol has been shown to have a detrimental effect on strength, power, endurance, coordination, reaction time, balance, and body temperature regulation. Ingestion after exercise can worsen dehydration, and slow down recovery and muscle repair. Alcohol is also an empty source of kilojoules and can lead to unwanted weight gain.

Tips for alcohol intake:
- Avoid alcohol in the 24 hours before competition.
- If you have any soft tissue injury or bruising, avoid alcohol in the 24-hour period after exercise.
- After exercise, rehydrate and refuel with carbohydrates before drinking alcohol.
- To reduce your intake, add plenty of ice or soda water to wine and spirits to dilute it, quench your thirst with non-alcoholic beverages first, or choose low-alcohol beer or wine.

**REHYDRATION**
Sports drinks can be an efficient source of hydration depending on the circumstances. Make your own using the recipes in this book.

# Increasing **Muscle Mass**

If you are involved in power sports such as rugby or sprinting, you may be regularly doing strength and resistance training to increase your muscle mass and improve your power-to-weight ratio (which means prioritizing gains in muscle mass without increasing fat mass).

In order to gain muscle mass effectively, a well-designed training programme (that includes both resistance exercise and a positive energy balance of at least 2,000–4,000 kJ (500–1,000kcal) per day) is required.

The following tips may help to increase your energy intake:

- Eat frequent meals and snacks throughout the day.
- Pack portable snacks if you have a busy day and/or are out and about (try cereal bars, dried fruit, or trail mix).
- Make use of energy-rich drinks such as smoothies, flavoured milk, or fruit juice.
- Limit your consumption of too many high fibre foods as these are more filling.
- Fortify foods to make them more energy rich. You can add skim milk powder, honey, fruit puree, or raisins to porridge; add extra layers of protein, healthy fats, and energy-rich carbohydrates to sandwiches (for example avocado and cheese; or peanut butter, banana, and honey).

It is important that carbohydrate supplies a significant amount of this energy, to provide fuel for the muscle to be able to do the training in order to stimulate growth.

## PACKING ON MUSCLE WITH PROTEIN

Your protein needs increase with strength training due to the synthesis of new muscle and supporting connective tissue, increased muscle hypertrophy and hypertrophy, and synthesis of enzymes needed for anaerobic metabolism to meet the energy demands of strength training. These increased protein needs are particularly high during the first 3–6 months of training due to muscle hypertrophy adaptations.

However, some studies suggest that as you become more trained, your body becomes more efficient at protein metabolism, which results in your body using less protein. In most instances, a high energy diet that provides 1.2–2g protein per kilogram body weight per day will be adequate to ensure that your protein needs are met. Consuming excess protein will not have extra anabolic effects. Overconsumption of protein will be used as fuel or contribute to gains in body fat. Very high protein intakes can also displace other important nutrients in your diet.

## TIMING OF PROTEIN INTAKE FOR MUSCLE GAIN

Your timing of protein intake may be just as important as your total protein intake over the day. If you consume large amounts of protein at one meal, only some of the protein will be used for muscle synthesis,

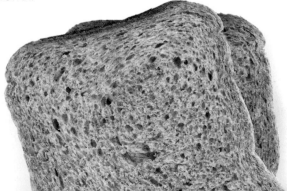

**BREAD**
You could eat a sandwich made with fresh wholegrain bread 3–5 hours before activity to meet your carbohydrate needs. Choose a low-fat filling.

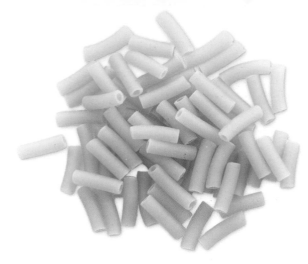

**PASTA**
Macaroni is a popular source of carbohydrates. Top it with cheese for a quick and simple protein boost.

and the rest will just result in increased protein use as fuel or body fat gain. Therefore, the most effective strategy for enhanced muscle hypertrophy and recovery is to include small amounts of protein at each meal and snack. Studies have shown that 20–25g of protein every 3–4 hours is optimal (for 85kg/187lb men doing resistance training). The addition of a bedtime snack consisting of protein and carbohydrate may also augment muscle protein synthesis.

Consuming a snack containing protein and carbohydrate before and immediately after resistance exercise can help to promote training adaptations by providing amino acids for muscle building, minimizing protein breakdown, and increasing the production of anabolic hormones. Snacks rich in carbohydrate and protein after training can also aid in the recovery of fuel stores. Post-exercise muscle protein synthesis is also enhanced by the inclusion of a protein rich in the amino acid leucine – a component of whey protein (found in dairy products).

Examples of recovery snacks:
- Flavoured milk or yogurt
- Smoothie with fruit and yogurt/milk
- Cereal and milk
- Lean meat/cheese sandwich

## SPORTS SUPPLEMENTS
There is a vast array of sports supplements, including protein powders, on the market that promise to increase muscle mass and strength. Most of these (expensive) supplements and their claims are not backed up with scientific evidence. This is because the supplement industry is poorly controlled globally and as a result many products are manufactured and sold without proof that they work. There may also be health and safety concerns with their use. Remember, that to get best results you need a properly designed training programme and a well-planned diet – supplements are not essential. If you still feel that your diet is not adequate and you would like to consider a supplement it is a good idea to seek expert advice from a registered dietitian or nutritionist working in sport before you make any decisions.

Look for recipes in this book with this icon, which signals a good source of protein.

**PROTEIN RICH**

# Controlling **Body Fat**

You may be aiming to lower your body fat or weight, particularly if you are an endurance athlete or involved in aesthetic sports such as gymnastics or ballet. However, it is important that you aim to do this in a safe manner in order to prevent adverse health issues and performance decline.

## SAFE WEIGHT LOSS

In order to lose weight effectively and safely, while still allowing enough energy to train optimally, you need to consider the following:

- Avoid quick-fix and fad diets, and adopt a balanced long-term strategy instead.
- If you have a lot of body fat to lose, take action during the off-season and not close to important events.
- Aim to lose no more than 0.5–1kg (1.1–2.2lb) body fat per week (or a maximum of 5mm / ¼in reduction in total skinfolds per week over 7 or 8 sites).
- Consult with a registered dietitian or nutritionist in order to develop a practical and individualised meal plan.

## DIETARY STRATEGIES TO LOWER BODY FAT

### Control portions and eat so that you stay fuller for longer

- Eat regularly to keep blood sugar levels stable and to prevent snacking on inappropriate foods.
- Fill up on "free" vegetables, for example broccoli, baby marrows, lettuce, cucumber, tomatoes, cauliflower, and peppers.
- Eat fresh fruit rather than drinking fruit juice.
- Choose wholegrain and lower GI carbohydrate-rich foods – these will help keep you fuller for longer.
- Add protein to meals so that they are more satiating.
- Buy pre-portioned snacks to avoid over-indulging.
- Reducing portion sizes when tapering or during the off-season.

### Plan ahead

- Use meals as post-recovery instead of having recovery snacks.
- Keep healthy food and snacks available, and keep unhealthy snacks out of sight.

### Manage social situations

- Make healthier choices when eating out. Try to avoid creamy sauces, or order salad dressings on the side.
- Choose a low-calorie starter such as a salad or non-creamy soup.
- Avoid buffets.
- Opt for fruit-based desserts.

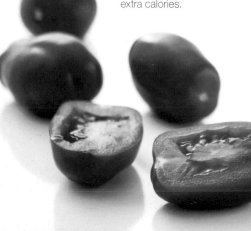

**ADD BULK TO MEALS**
Bulk up your meals with "free vegetables" to make them more filling without adding extra calories.

## Limit your fat intake

- Opt for healthier cooking methods (steaming, baking, grilling, and poaching).
- Avoid deep-fried and bread crumbed foods.
- Trim the fat off meat and the skin from chicken.
- Choose low-fat or fat-free dairy products.
- Choose snacks with <5g fat per 30g of carbohydrate.
- Choose low-fat sauces (for example tomato or vegetable-based instead of creamy sauces).
- Adapt recipes by using reduced-fat ingredients (low-fat plain yoghurt instead of cream; phyllo pastry instead of shortcrust pastry).

## Limit high-calorie and energy-dense foods and beverages

- Use refined carbohydrates such as sports drinks, soft drinks, sweets, and gels for prolonged, intense training sessions and competition purposes only.
- Drink mainly water instead of other beverages.
- If you really want something sweet to drink, dilute some fruit juice with water.
- Limit your alcohol intake.

## Increase your eating awareness

- Avoid sitting in front of the television or computer while eating. Sit at the table for meals.
- Eat slowly. It is a good idea to try put your knife and fork down between mouthfuls.
- Always plate your food and immediately pack leftovers away, out of sight. Never eat out of a box, packet, or carton.
- Savour every mouthful!
- Keep a food diary.

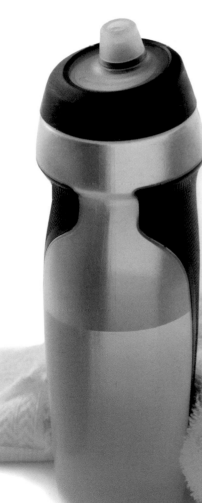

**DRINK MOSTLY WATER**
Limit the use of sports drinks and other sweetened beverages to prolonged intense training and competition.

# Eating for **Each Stage of Training**

**Your nutritional needs will be affected by your level of training and the stage you are at in the sport season. Many athletes break up a sport season into three phases: preparation, competition, and transition, with each phase having distinct goals and therefore requiring different nutrition strategies and amounts and ratios of nutrients.**

Nutrition periodization, or eating for each stage of training, is just as important as training periodization. To get the maximum benefit from training sessions, it is important to match your food intake to your fuel usage during training. Improper eating during hard training phases can lead to low energy stores and lower quality training sessions, while overeating during the off-season can lead to weight gain and increased body fat.

## NUTRIENT NEEDS FOR EACH STAGE OF TRAINING

Each athlete and sport will have different requirements in each stage, but from this example below you can see that carbohydrate and protein needs are usually higher during preparation and competition phases, whereas fat needs remains similar throughout. If you are training for ultra-endurance events your fat requirements may be higher.

| Phase | Carbs<br>Grams per kg<br>body weight | Protein<br>Grams per kg<br>body weight | Fat<br>% of daily total<br>energy intake |
| --- | --- | --- | --- |
| Preparation | 5–12 | 1.2–1.7 | 20–35% |
| Competition | 7–12 | 1.4–2.0 | 20–35% |
| Transition | 4–7 | 1.2–1.4 | 20–35% |

## THE PREPARATION PHASE

Your goal during this preparation phase might be to increase the intensity of your sport-specific training and increase your resistance training to build new muscle, improve strength and power, build up anaerobic conditioning, and tweak body fat levels. Training volume will most probably be higher.

Nutrition goals during this period include adequate carbohydrate and protein intake for supporting increased volume and intensity of training, building new muscle, and repairing damaged muscle. Nutrient-dense foods are important to ensure adequate intake of vitamins, minerals, and anti-oxidants.

This is also a good time to experiment with nutrition strategies, such as new products, timing of food intake, or nutrition levels during exercise.

## PREPARATION-PHASE NUTRIENT FOCUS

The following nutrients are essential for building endurance and intensity.

| | |
| --- | --- |
| Higher carbs | Fluids |
| Higher protein | Vitamins and minerals |

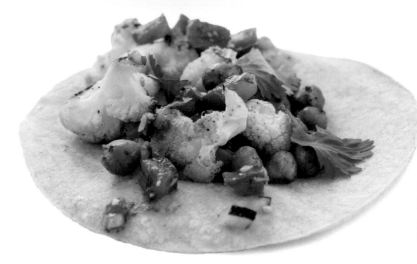

**POWER-PACKED CAULIFLOWER TACOS**
This portable, high-protein, high-carbohydrate dish is excellent for training days.

## THE COMPETITION PHASE

Your competition phase goals should be to maintain strength, power, and conditioning gains while continuing to improve performance. Resistance training may decrease during this phase with a focus on increasing exercise intensity while decreasing volume, adding core-strengthening activities, and focusing on injury prevention. Adequate recovery between competitions is important.

Your nutritional goals should focus on getting adequate carbohydrate, protein, fluids, vitamins, and minerals. It may be a good idea to limit high-fibre foods immediately before competition and straight afterwards, as they take longer to digest and may cause gastrointestinal complications and delay glycogen synthesis.

## THE TRANSITION PHASE

After the season is over, athletes typically go through a period of rest to allow their bodies to heal both physically and psychologically after the demands of the preparation and competition phases.

Recreational-type physical activity, such as squash, swimming, jogging, volleyball, and basketball, may be beneficial during this period of transition. The focus of this physical activity should be on lower intensities and decreased volume.

Nutritional needs decrease at this time, as should intake. Decrease your carbohydrate, protein, and fat intake to offset your decreased physical activity. Limit unintentional weight gain by decreasing portion sizes, eliminating additional snacking, and avoiding overconsumption of alcohol.

### COMPETITION-PHASE NUTRIENT FOCUS

Continue to get adequate carbs, protein, fluids, and vitamins and minerals, but limit fibre intake before activity.

| | |
|---|---|
| High carbs | Vitamins and minerals |
| High protein | Low fibre before exercise |
| Fluids | |

### TRANSITION-PHASE NUTRIENT FOCUS

Reduce your intake of carbohydrate and fat to avoid gaining weight due to your decreased activity.

| | |
|---|---|
| Adequate protein | Lower fat |
| Vitamins and minerals | Lower carbohydrate |

# The Vegan or **Vegetarian Athlete**

**Studies have shown that a well-planned vegetarian diet containing sufficient energy and protein, and which is low in fat with adequate carbohydrate, can be suitable for an athlete. It is important, however, that you, as a vegetarian or vegan athlete, are aware of potential dietary challenges.**

Vegan and vegetarian athletes may have to make more of an effort to meet overall calorie needs because many foods may be high in bulk and fibre.

Diets of vegetarians are often lower in protein than non-vegetarian diets, so athletes may need to be more conscious of targeting protein-rich vegetarian foods. Vegetable or plant proteins may be lacking in some essential amino acids, so will need to be combined in such a way that all essential amino acids are consumed. Thus it is important to include a variety of protein sources every day. Plant proteins are less well digested than animal proteins, so vegetarian athletes may need to aim to consume 10 per cent more protein than current sports protein recommendations.

Protein-rich plant based foods include legumes and beans (e.g. lentils, chickpeas, kidney beans, borlotti beans), soya, tempeh, tofu, textured vegetable protein, nuts, seeds, and grains. Energy-dense foods like nuts, tofu, tempeh, textured vegetable protein, cheese, and yoghurt, are low in bulk and can be incorporated into the diet especially when energy demands are high.

## TOP 5 VITAMINS AND MINERALS FOR VEGAN AND VEGETARIAN ATHLETES

Vegetarian and vegan athletes need to pay particular attention to the following vitamins and minerals:

**Vitamin $B_{12}$**   Necessary for red blood cell formation, neurological function, and DNA synthesis, vitamin $B_{12}$ is typically found in animal foods, but fortified breakfast cereals and grains, soya milk, and nutritional yeast products are also good sources. If you are a vegetarian athlete who consumes eggs and dairy products, you are likely to already meet $B_{12}$

requirements, but vegan athletes should ensure an adequate intake of $B_{12}$-fortified foods, or should take a $B_{12}$-containing multivitamin or supplement $B_{12}$ individually. Risks of inadequate $B_{12}$ intake include long-term damage due to neuropathy and anaemia.

**Calcium and vitamin D**   Inadequate calcium and vitamin D intake is associated with increased risk of stress fractures and decreased bone density. Weight-bearing physical activity helps to strengthen bones.

High-calcium plant-based foods include fortified orange juice; fortified cereals; almonds and almond butter; and green leafy vegetables, such as spinach, spring greens, broccoli, and Brussels sprouts. Dairy products (for vegetarians) or fortified milk alternatives, such as soya, rice, or almond milk, are also options.

The best source of vitamin D is from the sun. Most people need to spend 10–20 minutes in the sun every day at midday, with some skin exposed without sunscreen, in order to get enough. Athletes that are at higher risk for a deficiency are those who are older than 65, are dark-skinned, and who exercise indoors. There are few food sources – vegetarian sources include vitamin D fortified milk and margarine, as well as eggs (if chickens have been fed vitamin D) for ovo-vegetarians.

**Iron**   Many athletes are at an increased risk of iron-deficiency anaemia due to the inadequate intake of high-iron foods, iron losses via sweating, reduced absorption of iron, gastrointestinal bleeding, and (for women) menstrual blood loss. Iron is responsible for transporting oxygen in the body – without enough, athletic performance can be negatively affected. Haem sources of iron (like meat, chicken, and fish) are absorbed better than nonhaem sources (like spinach and legumes). Iron absorption can be inhibited by compounds in certain foods: polyphenols in cocoa and coffee; oxalates in tea, kale, beetroot, and chocolate; phytates in bran, nuts, seeds, and cereals. That said, there are some compounds that can enhance the absorption of nonhaem iron, specifically vitamin C.

A range of foods are good sources of iron, such as eggs (for ovo-vegetarians); fortified breakfast cereals; dark green leafy vegetables, such as kale and spinach (although iron may be poorly absorbed due to oxalates); beans, tofu, and soy beans; tempeh; enriched breads, rice and pasta; potatoes; quinoa; almonds; cashews; dried apricots and raisins; and blackstrap molasses.

**Zinc**   This mineral plays a role in several biochemical reactions and helps with proper function of the immune system. Zinc, like iron, is not absorbed as well due to higher concentrations of phytates. Vegetarian sources of zinc include hard cheeses, wheatgerm, Swiss chard, mushrooms, kidney beans, chickpeas, lentils, hummus, tofu, tempeh, peanut butter, nuts, and pumpkin and sunflower seeds.

**Omega-3 fatty acids**   These essential fatty acids cannot be synthesized by the body, so they must be obtained through dietary sources. Fish is typically a high source of omega-3. The best vegetarian sources of omega-3 include microalgae and sea vegetables. Flaxseeds (or linseeds), walnuts, and pumpkin and chia seeds all contain omega-3, but the bioavailability is poor.

Omega-3 fatty acids have many benefits, including reducing the risk of cardiovascular disease and helping decrease inflammation, which many athletes suffer from after physical activity or injury.

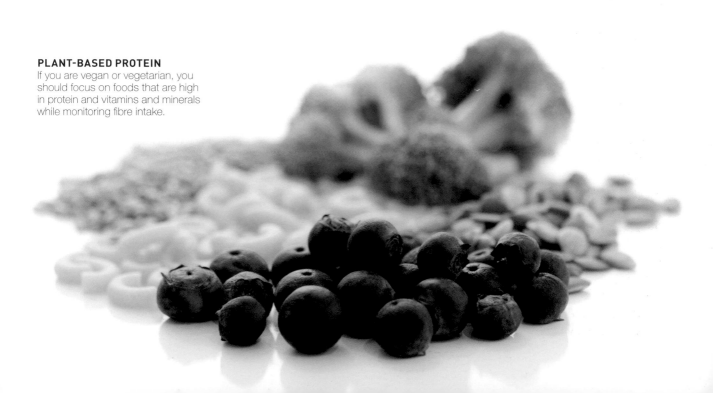

**PLANT-BASED PROTEIN**
If you are vegan or vegetarian, you should focus on foods that are high in protein and vitamins and minerals while monitoring fibre intake.

# Feeding a **Family of Athletes**

Feeding yourself, or an athlete in the family, is no easy task. You already have a packed schedule with your job or school, intense workouts, and competitions, and you still have to shop, and prepare meals within your budget. With homemade meals you are more in control of the nutritional content and you will most likely save money. In this section, we share a quick and easy weekly meal plan as well as tips on how to help implement it.

## MEAL PLANNING

Designate planning and shopping days. Pick one day of the week as your menu planning day, and another as your main food shopping day – but remember that you should shop for fresh produce 2–3 times a week. Look at your week's schedule and plan your meals and snacks for the week, taking into account particularly busy days, training sessions, how many you will be cooking for, and social events. Use the recipes provided, ideally incorporating at least two fish meals a week, 1-2 vegetarian meals, and a split

## SAMPLE ONE-WEEK MENU (Per Person)

| Meal | Sunday | Monday | Tuesday |
|---|---|---|---|
| Breakfast | 1 serving Blueberry Orange Parfaits | 1 serving Baked Country Ham, Egg, and Cheese Cups | 1 serving Cinnamon Crumble Muffins |
| Snack | 1 serving Apple Cinnamon Refresher | 240ml (8fl oz) low-fat Greek yogurt, 150g (5½oz) fresh berries | 75–100g (2½–3½oz) fresh vegetables, 4 tablespoons low-fat dip |
| Lunch (3 or 4 hours before training/competition) | 1 serving Turkey and Spring Onion Wraps, 1 small side salad | 1 serving Classic Chef Salad, 1 small roll | 1 serving Bean and Vegetable Soup, ½ sandwich |
| Snack (1 hour before training/competition) | 1 serving Sweet and Salty Peanut Bars | 30g (1oz) whole roasted almonds, 75g (2½oz) fresh strawberries | 240ml (8fl oz) low-fat Greek yogurt, 1 small plum |
| Training/Competition | 1 serving Gingerade | 1 serving Acai Punch | 1 serving Quick and Easy Energy Bars |
| Dinner (30 minutes to 1 hour after training/competion) | 1 serving Spicy Beef and Pasta Casserole, 1 side salad | 1 serving Garlic Chicken with Orzo Pasta, 1 side salad | 1 serving Slow Cooker Beef and Cabbage |
| Snack | 2 tablespoons peanut butter, 1 serving crackers | 1 serving Raisin and Bran Cookies | 150g (5½oz) mixed fruit |

between lean meat and chicken/turkey on remaining days. Use the sample one-week menu below to help get you started.

## CREATE A SHOPPING LIST

Check your cupboard for all the ingredients in the recipes and list those that you still need to purchase. If you notice you are running low on certain basic items, add these to your grocery list. Shopping from a list saves money and time – and limits impulse buying. You can also shop online (if available in your area).

## SHOPPING TIPS

Use your shopping list, and as far as possible try to buy produce that is locally sourced and in season. The best foods are those that will fuel your body as well as satisfy your taste buds. Limit your intake of processed foods. Be adventurous, and try new ingredients to spice up your routine. Keeping a variety of basic ingredients on hand will mean you are ready to tackle any recipe that sparks your interest.

Avoid shopping when hungry because this will prompt impulse buying – often of unhealthy foods.

| Wednesday | Thursday | Friday | Saturday |
| --- | --- | --- | --- |
| 1 serving Egg and Avocado Breakfast Burritos | 1 serving Green Monster Smoothie | 1 serving Orange Ginger Muffins | 1 serving Peaches and Cream Smoothie |
| 1 small banana, 30g (1oz) cashews | 1 serving Chocolate Peanut Butter Bars | 1 serving reduced-fat pretzels, 2 servings hummus | 30g (1oz) whole roasted almonds, 75g (2½oz) fresh blackberries |
| 1 serving Reduced-Fat Tuna Melts, 1 side salad | 1 serving Wholemeal Turkey and Veggie Pitta Sandwich, 1 serving Greek Pasta Salad | 1 serving lettuce salad, 240ml (8fl oz) chicken noodle soup | 1 serving Mediterranean Salmon Wraps, 150g (5½oz) diced fruit |
| 1 medium peach, 1 serving digestive biscuits | 1 medium apple, 2 tablespoons peanut butter | 75–100g (2½–3½oz) fresh vegetables, 4 tablespoons low-fat dip | 2 clementines, 60g (2oz) reduced-fat cheese |
| 1 serving Blackberry Cooler | 1 serving Cranberry Limeade | 1 serving Mango Cooler | 1 serving Lavender Lemonade Relaxer |
| 1 serving Stuffed Courgette Boats, 275g (11oz) rice | 1 serving Spaghetti with Meat Sauce, 1 small roll, 1 side salad | 1 serving Slow Cooker Pot Roast with vegetables | 1 serving Lentil Soup, 1 small roll, 1 side salad |
| 1 serving Strawberry Shortcake Milkshake | 180ml (6fl oz) reduced-fat frozen Greek yogurt, 30g (1oz) fresh blueberries | 1 serving Blueberry Madness Bars | 150g (5½oz) strawberries, 1 serving low-fat plain yogurt |

# Top 10 **Immune-Boosting Foods for Athletes**

To help fight infections, ensure your diet supplies sufficient energy, carbohydrate, protein, fat and micronutrients. Certain foods, with specific immune-boosting properties, should be eaten regularly.

Anti-oxidants are substances in food that can prevent or slow the oxidative damage to our body. They enhance our immune system and therefore lower the risk of infection. It is best to obtain antioxidants from a variety of foods instead of supplements.

**Green vegetables**   Green-coloured foods like broccoli and spinach contain antioxidants such as vitamins A and C, chlorophyll, isoflavones, and lutein. They also contain vitamin $B_6$, which can increase the production of immune fighting white cells.

**Blue and purple fruits and vegetables**   Blueberries, aubergines, and other blue- and purple-coloured foods contain the compounds quercetin, resveratrol, and anthocyanins, as well as vitamin C, which has antioxidant-like properties.

**Red coloured fruits and vegetables**   Foods such as red tomatoes, cherries, red peppers, beetroot, pomegranates, and watermelon contain lycopene, a phytonutrient with antioxidant-like properties. This has been associated with a decreased risk of cancers, including prostate, breast, and cervical.

**Yellow- and orange-coloured fruits and vegetables** Yellow- and orange-coloured foods contain beta-carotene, lycopene, potassium, and vitamins A and C. Try apricots, papaya, honeydew or cantaloupe melon, grapefruit, mangoes, nectarines, oranges, pumpkin, and sweet potatoes.

**Lean red meat**   This is a source of zinc, which is needed in several energy pathways in the body and to promote proper immune function. It also is a good

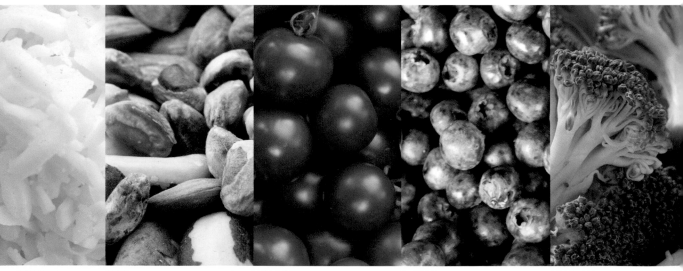

CHEESE    NUTS    TOMATOES    BLUEBERRIES    BROCCOLI

source of iron and vitamin $B_{12}$, both essential nutrients for optimal immunity. Choose lean cuts of meat and use low-fat cooking methods, such as grilling or frying in a non-stick pan with only a little oil.

**Fermented dairy products**    The probiotics that are found in fermented dairy products, such as probiotic-containing yogurt and kefir milk, are the first line of defence in our gut to protect against harmful bacteria. A bonus is that calcium – which is found in dairy products like yogurt and cheese – also ensures proper muscle function as well as helps to build strong bones.

**Sources of Omega 3**    Omega 3 fatty acids can help fight inflammation, and can therefore boost heart, brain, and joint health. It is commonly associated with fish, such as salmon, herring, mackerel, sardines, and tuna. Other sources of Omega 3 fatty acids include certain nuts, seeds, and oils.

**Ginger**    This spice contains phytochemicals and antioxidants that have been found to reduce inflammation. Ginger can be added to both sweet and savoury dishes, and features in many traditional cuisines, including Thai and Indian.

**Tea**    Flavonoids found in tea leaves act as strong antioxidants. They are water-soluble, which means that the longer you brew your cup of tea, the higher the amount of flavonoids that will be extracted. Although the chemical structure of flavonoids are different in black and green tea, the total amount of antioxidant activity remains similar. Aim, therefore, to drink up to 4 cups of unsweetened tea every day.

**Nuts**    Nuts are a great source of protein and vitamin E, which is important for cardiac health and as an antioxidant. Try raw or roasted nuts, such as cashews and walnuts, or spread nut butters, such as peanut butter or almond butter, on wholemeal bread or fruit as a snack.

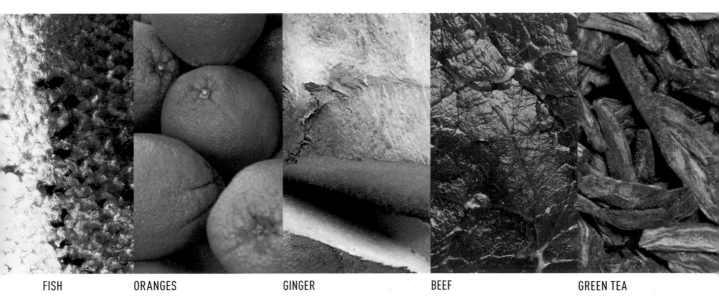

FISH          ORANGES          GINGER          BEEF          GREEN TEA

# Stocking **Your Kitchen**

Having a well-stocked kitchen is essential for quickly and easily preparing nutritious meals that can help to fuel your body. It will also prevent unnecessary trips to the grocery store, which will help you stick to your budget and save time.

## IN THE FRIDGE

**Vegetables and fruit**   Always have a variety of fresh and seasonal vegetables, salads, and fruit in your fridge.

**Meat**   Chicken, beef, pork, and seafood.

**Lean deli meats**   Turkey, chicken, or ham make for quick sandwich fillings or snacks. Look for cooked meats without (or with minimal) added preservatives or nitrites.

**Rotisserie chicken (preferably free range)**   This can be purchased already cooked at supermarkets. For a quick and easy meal, you can add the leftovers to soups, stews, or casseroles – or just to make a sandwich. Be sure to remove the skin.

**Dairy products**   Milk, yogurt, and cheeses. In addition to their carbohydrate and calcium component, milk and yogurt have the bonus of protein. Choose low-fat or reduced-fat items when appropriate.

## IN THE STORE CUPBOARD
### Protein

**Canned seafood**   Choose canned tuna, salmon, or shellfish, packed in water, brine, or tomato instead of oil to cut extra calories.

> **BE ORGANIZED**
> De-clutter your kitchen and clear out random items like magazines and keys that gather on surfaces but have nothing to do with food. By keeping your kitchen organized, you will know where everything is, and avoid wasting time looking for things. Ensure items used for food preparation are near to where you cook and easily accessible. Make sure to correctly store opened food packages to reduce spoilage, or use clear storage containers to enhance shelf life and make food in the cupboard more visible.

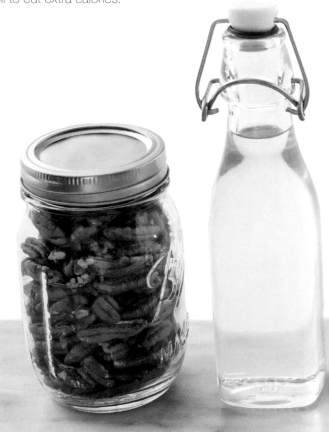

PECANS                    OLIVE OIL

**Canned beans**   These are a source of protein, fibre, and carbohydrate. Just drain and rinse, then you can add them to salads, soups, and casseroles, or enjoy them as a side dish. Good choices include black, cannellini, borlotti, and kidney beans, as well as chickpeas and lentils.

**Nuts and nut butters**   Almonds, walnuts, pecans, etc. Although these are high in fat, this is mostly healthy fat and they offer some protein as well.

## Carbohydrates

**Breads**   Wholemeal/wholewheat, seeded, rye, bagels, tortillas, pittas, and English muffins.

**Grains, seeds, and pastas**   Rice, barley, quinoa, oats, pasta, and couscous.

## Fruit and Vegetables

**Tomatoes (canned)**   Whole, chopped, purée, or sauce.

**Fruit (dried or canned in fruit juice)**   Peaches, pears, pineapple, apricots, cherries, and bananas.

**Potatoes**   Regular or sweet.

## Extras

**Oils**   Olive, rapeseed, avocado, and cooking sprays.

**Herbs and spices**   Oregano, basil, parsley, rosemary, cumin, bay leaves, thyme, coriander, tarragon, chives, dill, cinnamon, nutmeg, paprika, mustard, ginger, allspice, garlic, black pepper.

**Salt**   Salt comes in many different forms, but in the recipes in this book, we mostly use regular table salt.

**Baking ingredients**   Baking powder, bicarbonate of soda, cornflour, evaporated milk, vanilla extract, and dark chocolate chips.

**Condiments**   Tomato ketchup, mustard, and mayonnaise.

**Sauces**   Worcestershire sauce, hot pepper sauce, oyster sauce, and soy sauce.

**Vinegars**   White wine, apple cider, and balsamic.

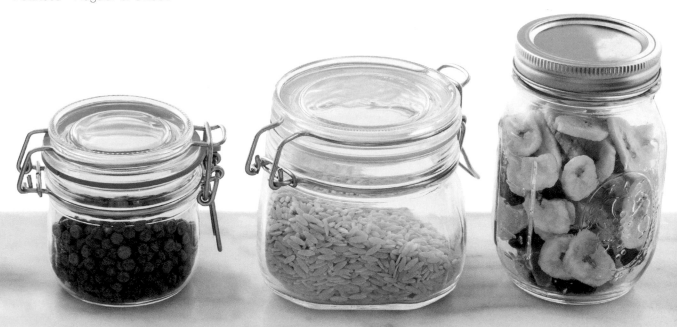

DARK CHOCOLATE CHIPS      ORZO PASTA      DRIED FRUIT

# Top 10 Kitchen Tools
# for Athletes

Having the proper utensils you need in the kitchen saves you time
and effort, and can prevent unnecessary injuries in the kitchen.

**1**

### MEASURING SPOONS AND JUGS
Every recipe requires precise
dry or liquid measurements.
Invest in a set of metal or plastic
measuring spoons for measuring
dry ingredients, and a measuring
jug for liquid ingredients.

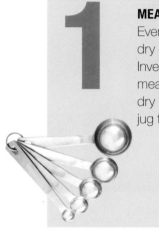

**2**

### BAKING TIN/CASSEROLE DISH
A 23 × 33cm (9 × 13in) dish
is great for making casseroles,
frittatas, and homemade baked
energy bars.

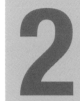

**3**

### KITCHEN SCALE
Ideal for measuring
ingredients accurately.

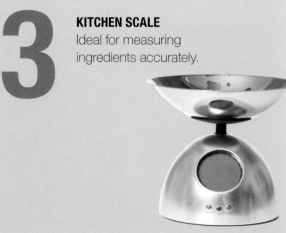

**4**

### FOOD PROCESSOR
This all-in-one versatile piece of
equipment can chop, slice, shred,
and purée, saving lots of time in
the kitchen.

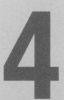

Other useful kitchen appliances and tools include a microwave, vegetable peeler and
slicer, tin opener, grater, garlic press, kitchen timer, thermometer, good mixing bowls,
colander, different size whisks, tongs, and heat-resistant spatulas.

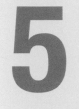

### 5 HAND-HELD OR STICK BLENDER

A blender is useful for making sports drinks, smoothies, milkshakes, fresh juice, salad dressings, and soups.

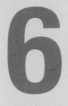

### 6 GOOD QUALITY CHOPPING BOARDS AND KNIVES

Save time and frustration with good quality chopping knives and boards. Having more than one chopping board can help to prevent cross-contamination. Essential knives to have include a chef's knife, paring knife, and a serrated knife. The handle should fit comfortably in your hand.

### 7 NONSTICK GRIDDLE OR FRYING PAN

Useful to quickly grill or stir-fry meat, chicken, fish, and vegetables with minimal oil. Consider buying dual purpose pans that can be used both on the hob and in the oven. Another good option is an electric non-stick griller – this handy appliance can bake or grill foods without needing to add additional fat.

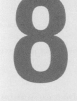

### 8 STEAMER

Various types of steamers are available, including microwave, bamboo, and stainless steel varieties. Quick way to prepare vegetables or fish.

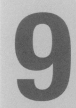

### 9 EGG BOILER/OMELETTE MAKER

Great for preparing breakfast-on-the-go, or even a light meal.

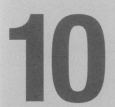

### 10 SLOW COOKER

This handy appliance cooks starters, meals, barbecue, chilli, soups, stews, side dishes, and even desserts over a longer period of time. Put ingredients into it in the morning, and come home after your workout to a ready meal.

# Quick-Cooking and Meal-Assembly Tips

Busy school, work, and training schedules mean there is not always a lot of time to spend in the kitchen. Here are some tips for making the most of your time while preparing wholesome food that will provide you with fuel.

## QUICK-COOKING METHODS

**Barbecueing**   Grilling cooks food quickly over high heat and adds flavour. Be sure to preheat the barbecue, whether it's a gas or charcoal one.

**Microwaving**   For heating leftovers and quick thawing. Many microwaves come with programmed times for commonly cooked foods.

**Stir-frying**   Cook small pieces of food quickly over high heat in a small amount of oil. The food must be constantly stirred to evenly distribute heat and avoid overcooking.

**Steaming**   This method of cooking is quick and generally healthier for you because it preserves nutrients better. By steaming vegetables you will lose less micronutrients compared to boiling them. Steaming within baking parchment parcels is another delicious way to prepare chicken, fish, and vegetables.

**Sautéing or pan-frying**   This high-heat cooking method is ideal for cooking meats and searing in juices. Remember to preheat the pan before adding oil, butter, or a cooking spray. Don't add additional foods too early, or the heat in the pan won't distribute evenly and food won't be cooked thoroughly. After sautéing meat, add a little bit of liquid, such as water or stock, to make a gravy.

**Grilling**   This method quickly cooks meats and vegetables. Remember to arrange the pan so that the food is the right distance away from the heat source.

**Pressure cooking**   This method cooks food quickly by increasing the pressure in the locked container and boiling the food at a high temperature. Most new models are digital and have safety features.

**Poaching**   Use liquid heated just under boiling point to simmer foods, such as eggs, fruits, and some meats.

**STIR-FRYING**
A fast and tasty way to cook protein foods and vegetables together, stir-frying gives you a super-satisfying meal.

**SLOW COOKING**
Although it's not quick per se, slow cooking is a time-saving cooking method for busy days. Simply toss everything in the slow cooker, set it to low, and your dish will be ready when you get home (usually in 6–8 hours).

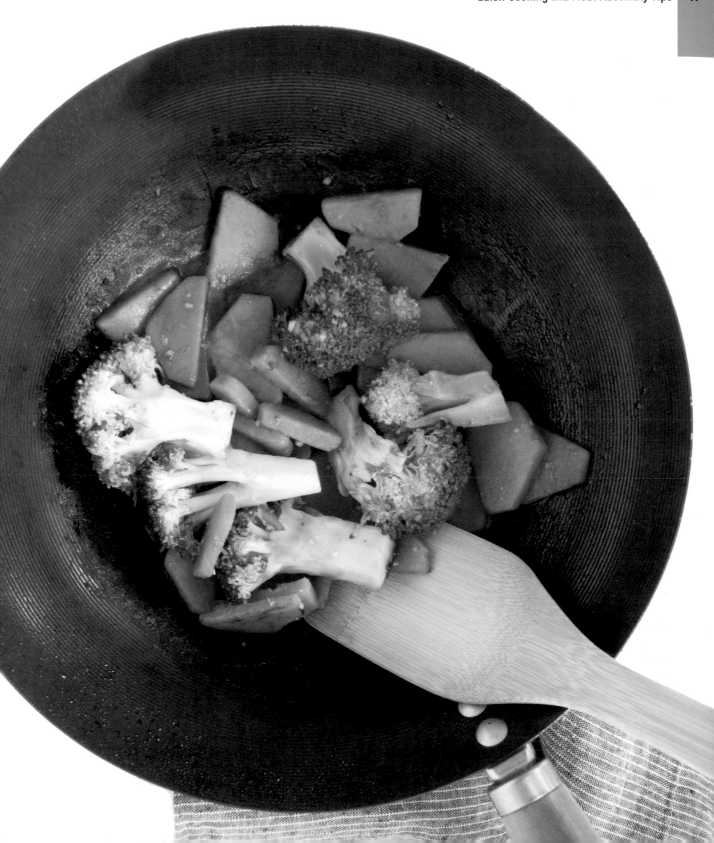

# Prepping **for Meals**

The French term *mise en place* means that you have all the ingredients measured out before starting to cook. This enables you to cook efficiently and without interruption. Here are some tips to help you get organized.

Before cooking make a rough mental (or physical) note of what you need to do by reading the recipe and checking you have all the ingredients you need. Remember to preheat the oven if needed.

A clean cook is an efficient cook. Always have a waste bowl next to you. It saves you going back and forth to the bin. Speed up clean-up by lining your baking dishes or trays with foil or baking parchment.

Ideally thaw frozen food by removing it from the freezer and thawing it in the fridge 12–24 hours before you need to use it.

Chop up fresh vegetables and store them in containers for quick use. You can also buy pre-cut vegetables, but they cost more. Chopped vegetables, such as onions, carrots, broccoli, cauliflower, and peppers store well in the fridge for several days. However, keep in mind that chopped vegetables will lose their nutritional value (particularly vitamins) and appearance much quicker. For best appearance and texture, wait until just before the meal to chop salad.

**PREPARED INGREDIENTS**
Use your prep day to chop vegetables, cook grains and pastas, or make sauces. Store them in separate containers in the fridge for later in the week.

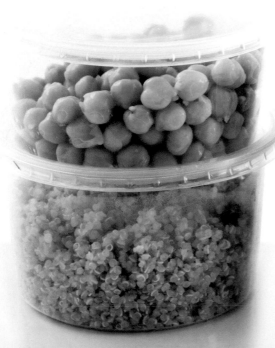
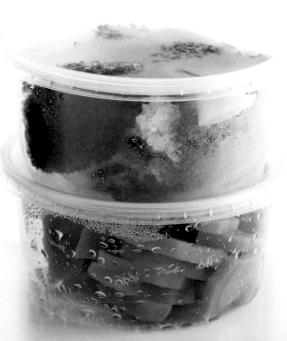

Cook big batches of minced meats such as beef, turkey, chicken, and hard-boiled eggs at the weekend to incorporate into meals throughout the week. Lean minced beef and minced turkey breast are perfect additions to sauces, soups, and chillis. Chicken can be sliced or diced and added to pasta, rice, soups, or salads. Hard-boiled eggs can be used sliced or chopped in salads or egg salad.

Cook large batches of grains and seeds, such as brown rice, barley, and quinoa. Use them within 3–4 days, or freeze for up to 1 month.

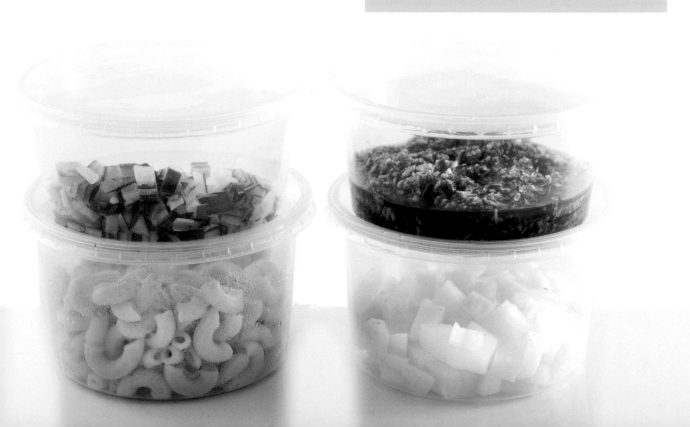

# Making **Portables**

**Healthy portable dishes – or portables – can play a big role in maintaining adequate nutritional intake. Distributing these calories throughout the day helps ensure your body has a steady stream of energy and is able to perform its best all day long.**

One of the most difficult things about being an athlete is maintaining adequate nutrition. You work out hard and burn extreme amounts of calories, so it is important that you make time to replenish your nutrition throughout the day.

Consuming regular meals throughout the day will help to ensure that you reach nutritional targets and that your body is being consistently nourished.

## WHAT ARE PORTABLES?

Most likely, you've been taking advantage of portables for a while now and might not even be aware that you are doing so. Portables can be any kind of foods that are easy to transport and can be held at room temperature (ideally) for pre-, mid-, or post-event snacks. Some portables you might be familiar with are cereal bars and trail mixes, etc.

Some portables are geared for different times in your workouts, so be sure to take a look at what you are eating so your body is able to get what it needs when it needs it.

In this book, we have three recipe sections, all of which contain recipes for various portables for different times in your workout – before, during, and after. We've put together some tasty, tested alternatives to shop-bought items, such as Baked Egg and Tomato Cups, Egg and Avocado Breakfast Burritos, and Mediterranean Salmon Wraps.

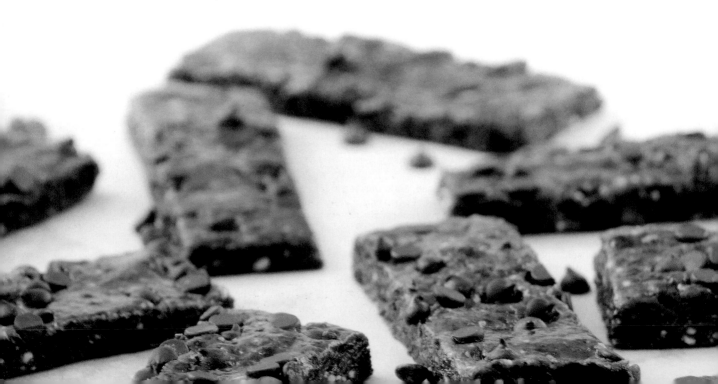

## MAKING PORTABLES TRANSPORTABLE

We've included a number of recipes for portables in this book, including energy bars, muffins, and wraps. To take these foods with you safely, be sure you wrap them well. Use zip-lock plastic bags for foods such as cookies, trail mixes, and other snacks; enclose items such as wrap-style sandwiches, baked egg cups, and muffins in baking parchment, foil, or cling film; or tuck some foods in reusable containers, such as salads, sandwiches, or other food items that may be a little messier with travel. Use whatever suits your situation best. Invest in good quality BPA-free plastic or glass containers. When heating food in the microwave, remember to decant into glass or porcelain.

In the recipes, we give suggestions on whether portables should be stored chilled or at room temperature for travel. Do not leave chilled items at room temperature for longer than 2 hours. Keep these recommendations in mind when choosing how to wrap your portables and how to best travel with them.

# Making Your Own **Sports Drinks and Smoothies**

**Sports drinks are an excellent way to replenish lost fluids, electrolytes, and carbohydrate used during a prolonged or intense workout. Smoothies replace fluids and can be a source of protein, carbohydrate, and other nutrients, so they are a good option for pre-event and recovery meals.**

The electrolyte content of sports drinks, particularly sodium, helps to preserve the thirst drive. Sodium concentrations of ~10Mm/L enhance the palatability and voluntary consumption of fluids consumed during exercise.

The taste and temperature of sports drinks are important factors as this will influence how much fluid is consumed. Generally you will drink more if you like the taste and if the drinks are cooler (especially in hot weather). Sports drinks can be served as an ice slurry both before and during exercise as part of a cooling strategy.

Homemade sports drinks and smoothies are a great alternative to commercially made versions. You can create flavour combinations that suit your tastes and adjust the nutrient content to fit your body's needs and avoid the colour additives and undesirable preservatives often found in shop-bought drinks. In addition, creating your own sports drinks and smoothies can keep your costs down.

**DIY sports drinks**   You can prepare these sports drinks ahead of time and store them in bottles, jugs, flasks, etc. until you are ready to drink them.

Be aware that sports drinks (and other carbohydrate containing fluids like fruit juice and soft drinks) can contribute to dental erosion. It is therefore important to:

- Limit contact of these drinks with teeth. Do not swish drinks around your mouth.
- Use a straw or squeezy bottle.
- Chew sugar-free gum or consume a dairy product after drinking a sports drink.

The type and quantity of carbohydrates provided in sports drinks varies. When choosing a drink, take into consideration your personal goal and factors such as taste, situations for use, and gut tolerance.

It is important to note that you need to take into account your body composition goals, age and nutritional goals when deciding whether to consume sports drinks. Sports drinks are not needed at every training session. Drinking too much energy-dense fluids such as sports drinks will increase energy intake and can lead to unwanted weight gain. On some occasions you maybe deliberately choose to not consume a sports drink during a session to increase the adaptive response to exercise. For more information, check out **Train Low, Compete High** on page 20.

## COMMON DRINKS AND THEIR CONCENTRATIONS

| PERCENTAGE | USE | EXAMPLES |
|---|---|---|
| <5.9% (0-5.9g/100ml) | These drinks are useful when hydration needs are greater than fuel needs, short training sessions (<60min), and/or when total calories need to be limited to prevent weight gain (e.g. gymnasts and weight lifters). In some cases they are sweetened in part or entirely with artificial sweeteners for taste, so as to encourage fluid consumption. | • Powerade Zero<br>• Lucozade Sport Lite<br>• PowerBar Isolite |
| 6-8% (6-8g/100ml) | These are designed to replace fluid lost from sweat, as well as provide carbohydrate for energy. The concentration has been shown to be the most ideal concentration for rapid delivery of fluid and fuel, and to maximise gastric tolerance and palatability. Useful for endurance athletes, or those who need both fluid and carbohydrate in their daily workout routine. | • PowerBar Isomax (50g/750ml)<br>• Lucozade Sport<br>• Isostar<br>• Powerade Isotonic<br>• Gatorade |
| >8% (>8g/100ml) | These drinks contain high concentrations of carbohydrate and are used to maintain muscle glycogen stores. They can be useful before or after training for athletes who have very high calorie and carbohydrate requirements e.g. Ironman triathletes. These are not suitable during high intensity exercise as they may result in gastrointestinal upset. | • Powerbar Isomax (50g per 500ml)<br>• High 5 EnergySource<br>• Commercial ice tea<br>• Coca-Cola<br>• 100% fruit juice |

## SENSATIONAL SMOOTHIES

Smoothies are a superb option for packing fruits, vegetables, calories, protein, and plenty micronutrients into your diet, depending on what you need for your specific workout. They can be prepared quickly and easily with just a little planning and preparation.

The best advantage of drinking a smoothie is that you can get in all the macro- (carbohydrate, protein, and fat) and micronutrients (vitamins and minerals) you need without having to consume lots of solid food – great if you have a low appetite.

The typical smoothie starts with a base, such as low-fat plain yogurt, milk, or soya milk. Add to that fruits, such as bananas for a smoother consistency, strawberries for taste and fibre, and oranges for vitamin C.

You also can add powerful vegetables, such as spinach, broccoli, or kale, and you will hardly notice them. Add some nuts or seeds for extra texture and protein, and include some ice.

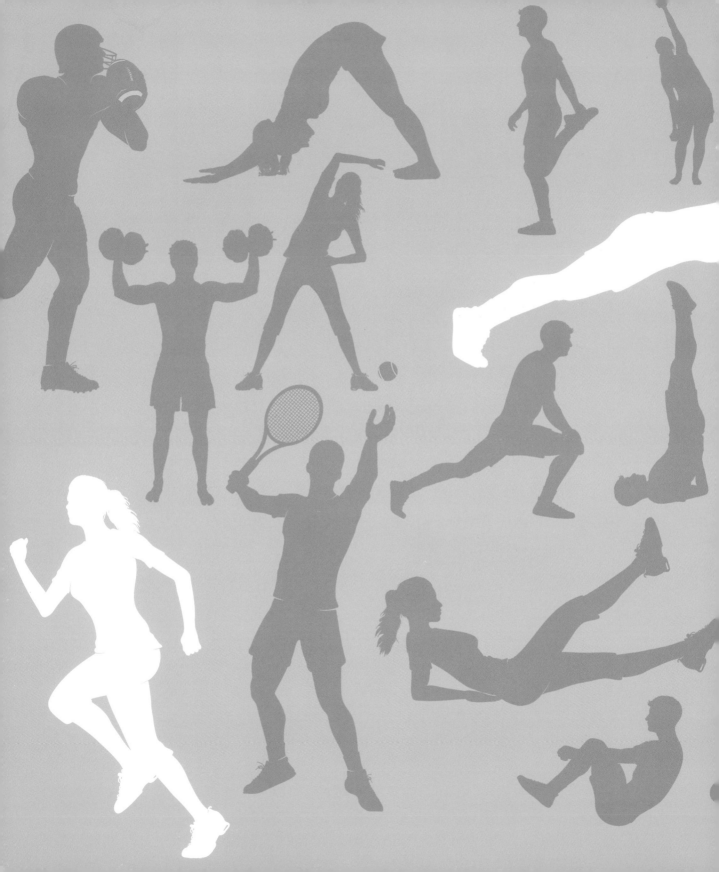

# Recipes for
# **Training**

In Part 2 we have brought together the nutritional principles from the previous sections in the form of easy-to-prepare recipes from homemade sports drinks and smoothies to delicious portable meals, soups, salads, mains, and desserts.

These recipes have been designed to help keep your nutritional goals in check by incorporating a variety of carbohydrate-rich foods (cereals; grains; fruit and starchy vegetables), as well as lean protein-rich foods (fish; lean meat; lean ham, skinless chicken; eggs; low fat dairy) and food rich in healthy fats (olive oil, avocado pear, hummus).

Take note that some recipes in this section may cause gastro-intestinal discomfort such as bloating if consumed shortly before (2–4 hours) or during training. Experiment with the timing of these meals to see what you tolerate the best.

**Note** Low fat yogurt refers to 1.5g fat/100ml

2

# Cranberry
# **Limeade**

Cranberry and lime juices combine with the sweetness of fresh orange juice in this bubbly thirst-quencher that is high in vitamin C. Contains 9g carbohydrate/100ml.

● ● ● **Easy**

**PREP** 5 mins

**SERVES** 1

## INGREDIENTS

1 tbsp lime cordial
2 tbsp fresh orange juice
120ml (4fl oz) cranberry juice
180ml (6fl oz) water
½ tsp salt

1 Combine all the ingredients together in a water bottle and mix.

2 Consume chilled or over ice.

| NUTRITION PER SERVING | |
|---|---|
| ENERGY | 546kJ (130kcal) |
| CARBOHYDRATES | 32g |
| SUGARS | 29g |
| DIETARY FIBRE | 0g |
| PROTEIN | 0g |
| FAT | 0g |
| CHOLESTEROL | 0g |
| SODIUM | 290mg |
| VITAMIN C | 90% |
| VITAMIN A | 10% |
| IRON | 6% |

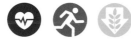

# Coco Melon Lime
# **Cooler**

This refreshing drink is ideal if you have high energy requirements and your gut can tolerate fructose during training. The watermelon is a source of the antioxidant vitamins A and C, and counts towards one of your 5-a-day fruit servings.

● ● ● **Easy**

**PREP** 5 mins

**SERVES** 1

## INGREDIENTS

220g (7½oz) cubed watermelon
240ml (8fl oz) coconut water
Juice of ¼ lime (about 1½ tsp)

1 Combine all the ingredients together in a blender, and whizz until smooth.

2 Drink immediately.

| NUTRITION PER SERVING | |
|---|---|
| ENERGY | 496kJ (118kcal) |
| CARBOHYDRATES | 23.6g |
| SUGARS | 22.8g |
| DIETARY FIBRE | 2.6g |
| PROTEIN | 2.5g |
| FAT | 0.2g |
| CHOLESTEROL | 0g |
| SODIUM | 71mg |
| VITAMIN C | 39% |
| VITAMIN A | 24% |
| IRON | 3% |

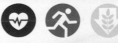

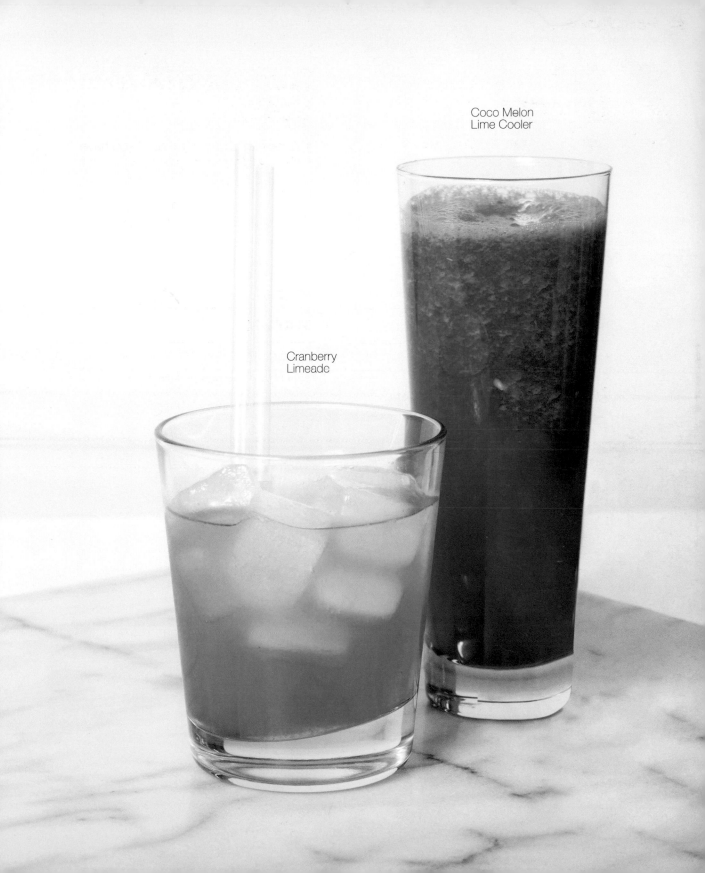

Coco Melon
Lime Cooler

Cranberry
Limeade

# Blackberry
## Cooler

Use still water instead of sparkling in this antioxidant-rich drink to reduce the risk of gastro-intestinal discomfort when consumed just before or during training.

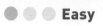 **Easy**

**PREP** 5 mins

**SERVES** 1

### INGREDIENTS

4 fresh mint leaves
5 fresh blackberries
2 tsp honey
Juice of ½ lemon (about 1 tbsp)
120ml (4fl oz) sparkling water
60ml (2fl oz) coconut water

**1** In a large glass, combine the mint and blackberries. Crush the blackberries with the back of a spoon.

**2** Stir in the honey, lemon juice, sparkling water, and coconut water. Enjoy immediately.

### NUTRITION PER SERVING

| ENERGY | 378kJ (90kcal) |
|---|---|
| CARBOHYDRATES | 23g |
| SUGARS | 16g |
| DIETARY FIBRE | 5g |
| PROTEIN | 2g |
| FAT | 0g |
| CHOLESTEROL | 0g |
| SODIUM | 65mg |
| VITAMIN C | 50% |
| VITAMIN A | 4% |
| IRON | 4% |

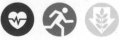

# Acai
## Punch

Look for 100% acai juice that contains no added preservatives. Note: allergic reactions can occur if you have a pollen allergy or sensitivity to the acai palm.

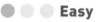 **Easy**

**PREP** 5 mins

**SERVES** 1

### INGREDIENTS

4 fresh mint leaves
⅛ tsp salt
2 lime wedges
180ml (6fl oz) acai juice
90ml (3fl oz) water

**1** In a large glass, combine the mint, salt, and lime wedges, and press together with the back of a spoon until the salt starts to dissolve in the juice.

**2** Pour in the acai juice and water, and combine. Enjoy immediately over ice.

### NUTRITION PER SERVING

| ENERGY | 378kJ (90kcal) |
|---|---|
| CARBOHYDRATES | 21g |
| SUGARS | 20g |
| DIETARY FIBRE | 0g |
| PROTEIN | 0g |
| FAT | 0g |
| CHOLESTEROL | 0g |
| SODIUM | 55mg |
| VITAMIN C | 130% |
| VITAMIN A | 0% |
| IRON | 8% |

# Super-Easy
## Sports Drink

Diluting the fruit juice and adding sugar improves the fructose to glucose ratio so the carbs are better used.

**Easy**

**PREP** 2 mins

**SERVES** 12

### INGREDIENTS

1.5 litres (2¾ pints) any flavour of juice
1.5 litres (2¾ pints) water
2 tbsp sugar
½ tsp salt

**1** Combine all the ingredients together in a large jug.

**2** Refrigerate for up to 1 week.

### NUTRITION PER SERVING

| ENERGY | 328kJ (78kcal) |
|---|---|
| CARBOHYDRATES | 18.9g |
| SUGARS | 2.5g |
| DIETARY FIBRE | 0.1g |
| PROTEIN | 0.1g |
| FAT | 0g |
| CHOLESTEROL | 0g |
| SODIUM | 83mg |
| VITAMIN C | 46% |
| VITAMIN A | 0% |
| IRON | 0% |

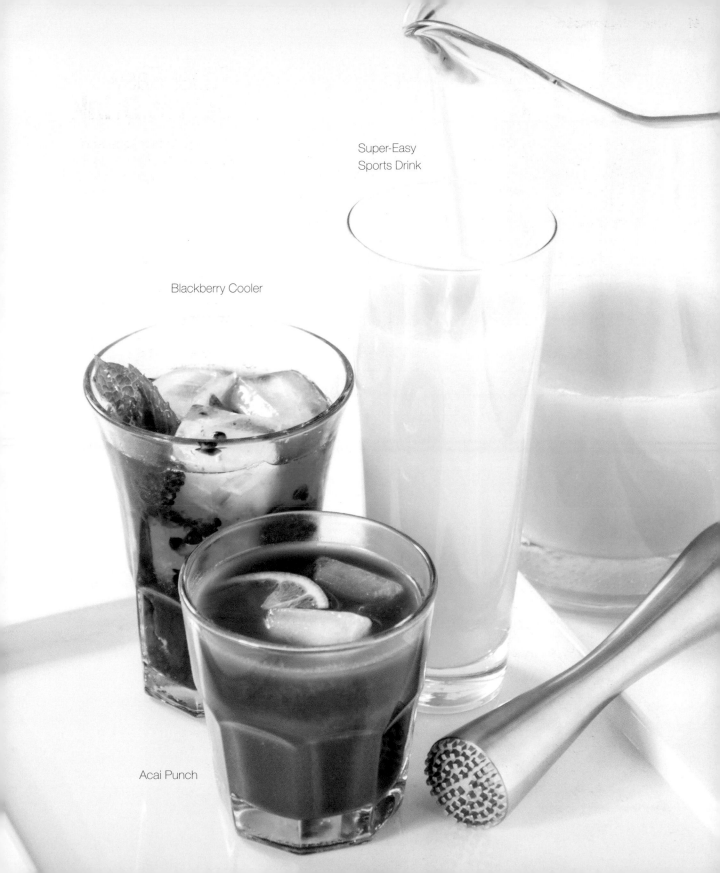

Super-Easy
Sports Drink

Blackberry Cooler

Acai Punch

# Baked Ham, Egg, and Cheese **Cups**

This convenient, protein-rich recipe can be baked ahead of time and eaten on the go. Serve with a toasted English muffin and some fruit for a complete meal.

● ○ ○    **Easy**

**PREP** 10 mins
**COOK** about 45 mins

**MAKES** 12

## INGREDIENTS

1 medium sweet potato, washed, peeled, and shredded

1 tsp extra-virgin olive oil

½ tsp sea salt

¼ tsp freshly ground black pepper

12 large eggs

110g (scant 4oz) dry-cured ham, such as Parma or proscuitto, roughly chopped

115g (4oz) sharp Cheddar cheese, grated

You can easily adapt this base recipe to suit your tastes: replace ham with smoked salmon, or turn it into a vegetarian option by replacing the ham with spinach and goat's cheese.

1 Preheat the oven to 180°C (350°F/gas 4). Lightly grease a 12-hole muffin tin with cooking spray.

2 In a small bowl, combine the sweet potato with the olive oil, sea salt, and black pepper.

3 Evenly divide the sweet potato mixture between the holes of the muffin tin and pat down a bit to make a crust.

4 Bake the sweet potato mixture for 15–20 minutes, or until the sweet potato starts to brown.

5 Remove the muffin tin from the oven, and crack 1 egg into each hole. Evenly distribute the chopped ham and cheese over the top of each egg.

6 Return the muffin tin to the oven for 20–25 minutes, or until the eggs are firm.

7 Allow eggs to cool to room temperature before serving.

8 Store leftovers in a zip-lock plastic bag in the fridge or freezer. Reheat in the oven or microwave when needed.

**Make ahead and freeze:** Refrigerate after step 8 for up to 5 days, or freeze for up to 2 months.

| NUTRITION PER SERVING | | | |
|---|---|---|---|
| ENERGY | 462kJ (110kcal) | FAT | 6g |
| CARBOHYDRATES | 3g | CHOLESTEROL | 220mg |
| SUGARS | 1g | SODIUM | 440mg |
| DIETARY FIBRE | 1g | VITAMIN C | 2% |
| PROTEIN | 11g | VITAMIN A | 45% |
| | | IRON | 6% |

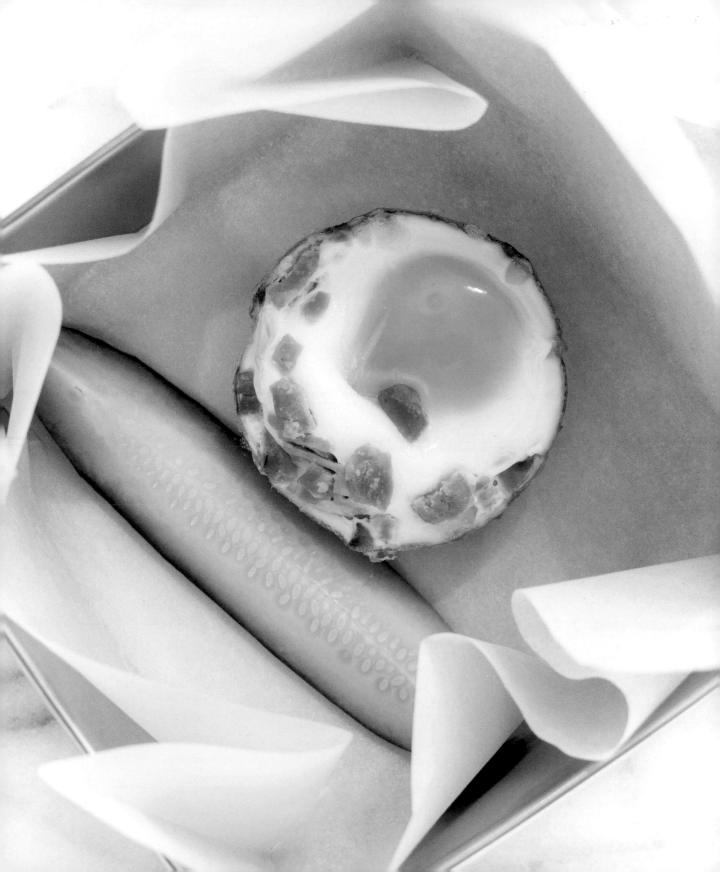

# Egg and Avocado
# **Breakfast Burritos**

Make these burritos ahead of time and eat them cold, or reheat them in the microwave if you prefer. They are a source of protein, while the avocado also provides some healthy fat.

● **Easy**

**PREP** 5 mins
**COOK** 7 mins

**SERVES** 4

## INGREDIENTS

6 large eggs

1 tbsp extra-virgin olive oil

¼ medium red onion, finely diced (about 45g [1½oz])

4 x 15cm (6in) wheat tortillas

4 tbsp salsa

2 small avocados, peeled, stoned, and sliced

Fresh coriander, to garnish (optional)

1 In a medium bowl, whisk together the eggs. Set aside.

2 In a frying pan over a medium–low heat, heat the oil and sauté the red onion for 1–2 minutes, or until softening.

3 Pour the eggs into the frying pan, and scramble for 4–5 minutes, or until the eggs are cooked through.

4 Evenly divide the egg mixture between the 4 tortillas, and top each serving with 1 tablespoon of salsa and sliced avocado (about ½ avocado for each).

5 Garnish with a few coriander leaves, if desired, and roll the tortillas around the filling. Serve on the same day.

To make this recipe higher in fibre, use whole wheat tortillas. For an extra kick add pickled jalapeños.

| NUTRITION PER SERVING | | | | |
|---|---|---|---|---|
| ENERGY | 1,890kJ (450kcal) | FAT | 6g |
| CARBOHYDRATES | 34g | CHOLESTEROL | 315mg |
| SUGARS | 4g | SODIUM | 370mg |
| DIETARY FIBRE | 9g | VITAMIN C | 35% |
| PROTEIN | 16g | VITAMIN A | 10% |
| | | IRON | 15% |

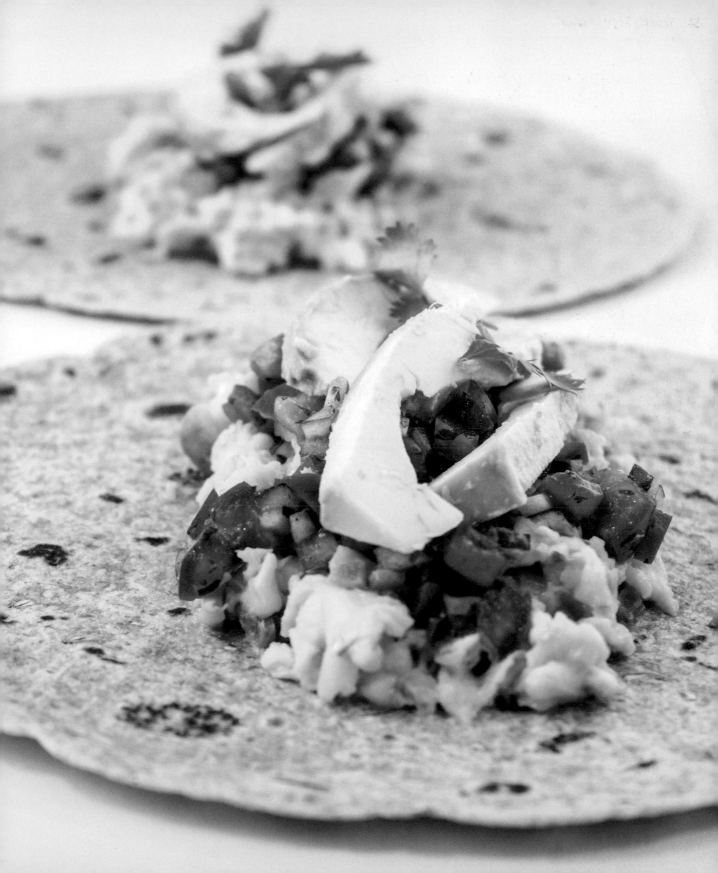

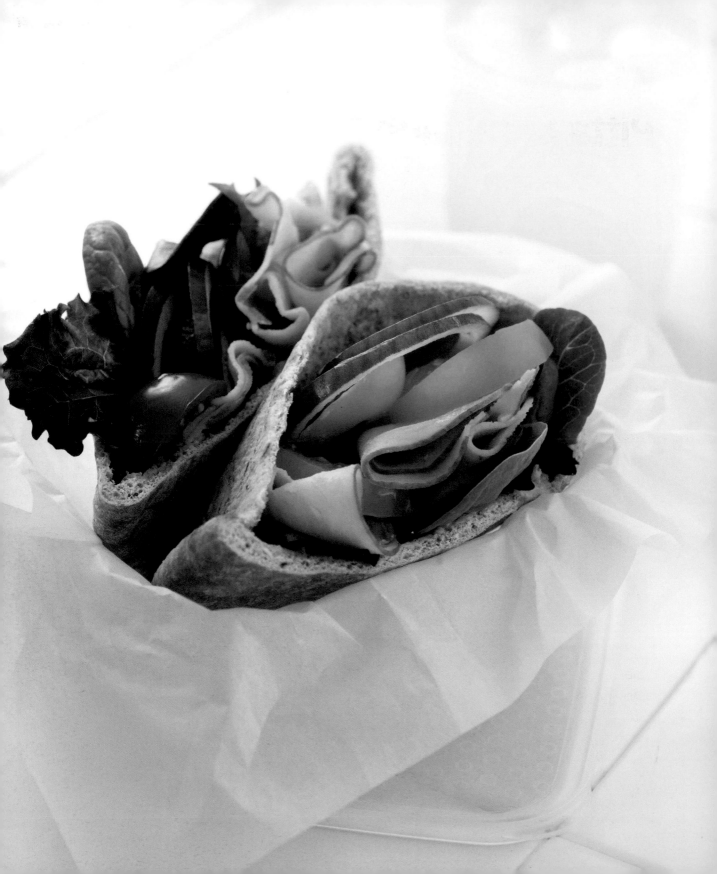

# Wholemeal Turkey and Veggie
# **Pitta Sandwich**

These pitta pockets are a great light lunch option. Not only does this sandwich travel well, but it also provides a balanced meal of protein, carbohydrate, fibre and healthy fats.

1  Halve the pitta and spread the hummus inside each half.

2  Fill the pitta with turkey breast, lettuce leaves, tomato slices, cucumber slices, and red onion slices.

3  Enjoy immediately or wrap up and take for your lunch.

● **Easy**

**PREP** 5 mins

**SERVES** 1

**INGREDIENTS**

1 x 16.5cm (6½in) wholemeal pitta

2 tbsp hummus

60g (2oz) cooked turkey breast slices

Handful lettuce leaves

1 small tomato, sliced

4 slices cucumber

2 slices red onion

| NUTRITION PER SERVING | | | |
|---|---|---|---|
| ENERGY | 1,243kJ (296kcal) | FAT | 6.5g |
| CARBOHYDRATES | 41g | CHOLESTEROL | 29mg |
| SUGARS | 2g | SODIUM | 430mg |
| DIETARY FIBRE | 7.2g | VITAMIN C | 9% |
| PROTEIN | 21g | VITAMIN A | 2% |
| | | IRON | 26% |

Use any leftover protein such as chicken or steak, or swap the hummus for ¼ avocado (25g). If you would like to reduce the fibre for a pre-training meal, use white pitta bread.

# Sweet and Salty **Peanut Bars**

Packed with dates, peanut butter, and heart-healthy oats, these are an excellent source of healthy fats. Ditch the shop-bought snacks.

 **Easy**

**PREP** 10 mins
**COOK** 25–30 mins

**MAKES** 10

## INGREDIENTS

175g (6oz) dried dates, pitted and finely chopped

125g (4½oz) crunchy peanut butter

100g (3½oz) rolled oats

2 tbsp honey

**1** Line a 20 × 20cm (8 × 8-in) cake tin or baking tray with baking parchment.

**2** In a food processor, combine the dates, peanut butter, rolled oats, and honey, then pulse until well combined.

**3** Press the mixture into the bottom of the prepared tin or dish, and refrigerate for 25–30 minutes.

**4** When the mixture has hardened, remove from the tin or dish and cut into 10 evenly sized bars. Store leftovers in a zip-lock plastic bag or other airtight container.

**Make ahead and freeze:** Prepare up to step 4, store in an airtight container at room temperature or refrigerate for up to 1 week; freeze for up to 1 month.

Replace peanut butter with any other nut butter such as almond or macadamia butter.

| NUTRITION PER SERVING | | | |
|---|---|---|---|
| ENERGY | 825kJ (196kcal) | FAT | 7.4g |
| CARBOHYDRATES | 25g | CHOLESTEROL | 0mg |
| SUGARS | 12g | SODIUM | 62mg |
| DIETARY FIBRE | 3g | VITAMIN C | 0% |
| PROTEIN | 4.5g | VITAMIN A | 0% |
| | | IRON | 6% |

# Tropical Island **Trail Mix**

A tasty and portable snack to help meet high energy requirements. Make a batch of this mix, divide into serving sizes, and store in small containers or zip-lock bags that you can keep on hand for a super-quick, healthy snack at any time of the day.

1. In a large bowl, simply toss together all of the ingredients until well combined.

2. Store in an airtight container, or divide into 12 small snacking bags.

**Make ahead:** Store in an airtight container at room temperature for up to 2 weeks.

● **Easy**

**PREP** 5 mins

**MAKES** 12 portions

### INGREDIENTS

50g (1¾oz) raw almonds
50g (1¾oz) raw Brazil nuts
30g (1oz) roasted hazelnuts
30g (1oz) roasted pumpkin seeds
60g (2oz) dried banana chips
60g (2oz) dried pineapple chunks
60g (2oz) dried papaya chunks
20g (¾oz) coconut chips
1 tsp ground cinnamon

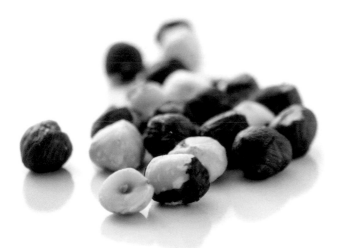

### NUTRITION PER SERVING

| | | | |
|---|---|---|---|
| **ENERGY** | 911kJ (217kcal) | **FAT** | 14.6g |
| **CARBOHYDRATES** | 15.4g | **CHOLESTEROL** | 0mg |
| **SUGARS** | 10g | **SODIUM** | 20.3mg |
| **DIETARY FIBRE** | 4.7g | **VITAMIN C** | 0% |
| **PROTEIN** | 4.1g | **VITAMIN A** | 0% |
| | | **IRON** | 0% |

To lower the saturated fat content, omit the coconut chips. If you prefer, you can replace the tropical dried fruit in this recipe with 160g (5¾oz) dried berry mix. Look out for unsulphured dried fruit.

# Blueberry Madness **Bars**

These bars are a chewy treat. They contain healthy fats and antioxidants, and are lower in sugar than shop-bought alternatives.

● ● ○    **Intermediate**

**PREP** 15 mins
**COOK** 50 mins

**MAKES** 12

## INGREDIENTS

65g (2oz) brown sugar
1 tsp baking powder
125g (4½oz) plain flour
¼ tsp salt
½ tsp ground cinnamon
60g (2oz) rolled oats
90ml (3fl oz) rapeseed oil
2 tbsp unsweetened apple sauce
1 large egg
3 tsp cornflour
500g (1lb 2oz) fresh blueberries
2 tbsp sugar

**Crumb topping**
30g (1oz) brown sugar
1 tsp ground cinnamon
¼ tsp salt
2 tbsp canola oil
30g (1oz) plain flour
15g (½ oz) wholemeal flour
15g (½ oz) rolled oats

If you can't find fresh blueberries, you can use frozen mixed berries instead (just remember to defrost before use).

1 Preheat the oven to 190°C (375°F/gas 5). Lightly grease a 23 × 33cm (9 × 13in) baking tray.

2 In a medium bowl, combine the sugar, baking powder, flour, salt, and cinnamon. Stir the rolled oats into the flour mixture until evenly distributed.

3 Mix the oil, apple sauce and egg and add to the dough.

4 Press three-quarters of the dough mixture into the prepared baking tin (using your hands works best).

5 In a separate bowl, stir together the remaining sugar and cornflour. Gently fold in the blueberries, and then pour this blueberry mixture over the dough layer.

6 Mix together the crumb ingredients and sprinkle over the top.

7 Bake for 45–50 minutes, or until the top is lightly golden brown.

8 Allow to cool completely before cutting into 12 bars.

**Make ahead and freeze:** Prepare up to step 8, store in an airtight container at room temperature for up to 3 days, refrigerate for up to 1 week, or freeze for up to 1 month.

| NUTRITION PER SERVING | | | |
|---|---|---|---|
| ENERGY | 926kJ (229kcal) | FAT | 9.7g |
| CARBOHYDRATES | 30.4g | CHOLESTEROL | 17mg |
| SUGARS | 5.3g | SODIUM | 103mg |
| DIETARY FIBRE | 2.2g | VITAMIN C | 7.5% |
| PROTEIN | 2.8g | VITAMIN A | 0% |
| | | IRON | 7% |

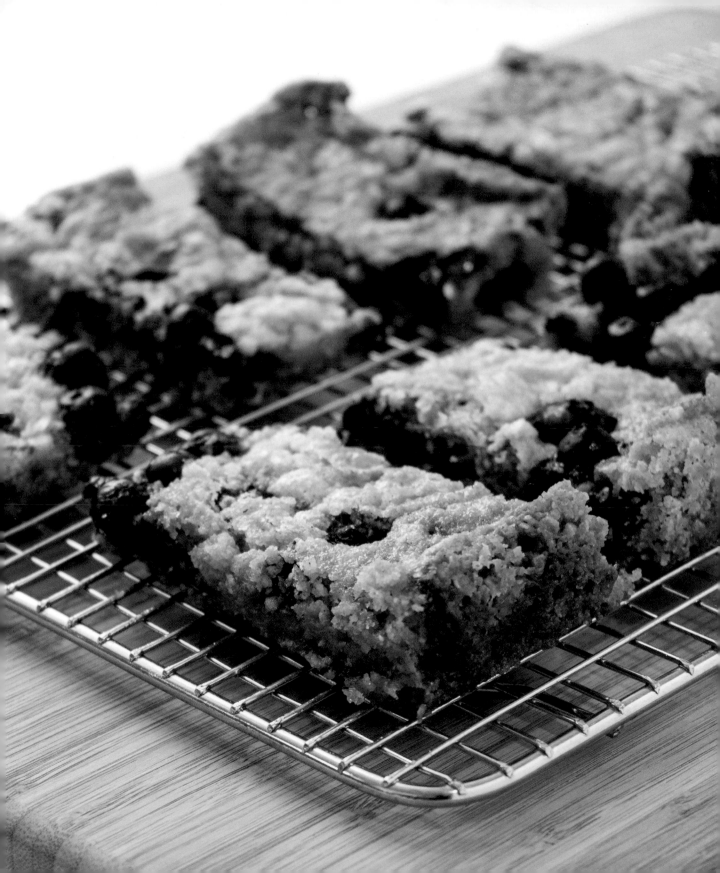

# Cinnamon **Crumble Muffins**

These muffins are made with wholemeal flour and healthy oils and are topped with a delicious and crunchy crumb topping. Store leftover muffins in an airtight container.

● ● **Intermediate**

**PREP** 10 mins
**COOK** 15–17 minutes + cooling

**MAKES** 6 large muffins

## INGREDIENTS

**Crumb topping**
30g (1oz) brown sugar
1 tsp ground cinnamon
¼ tsp salt
30ml (1fl oz) rapeseed oil
30g (1oz) plain flour
15g (½oz) wholemeal flour
15g (½oz) rolled oats

**Muffin mixture**
125g (4½oz) plain flour
60g (2oz) wholemeal flour
85g (3oz) brown sugar
2 tsp baking powder
1 tsp ground cinnamon
¼ tsp bicarbonate of soda
¼ tsp salt
180ml (6fl oz) skimmed milk
2 tbsp olive oil
2½ tbsp unsweetened
   apple sauce
3 egg whites

For more fibre, replace the white flour with wholemeal.

1 Preheat the oven to 190°C (375°F/gas 5). Line a 6-hole muffin tin with paper cases or coat with cooking spray.

2 *For crumb topping:* in a medium bowl, combine the sugar, cinnamon, and salt. Add in the oil until combined.

3 Add the flours and rolled oats, and stir using a spoon or rubber spatula until the mixture becomes moist. Spread out the mixture on the bottom of the bowl and set aside.

4 *For muffins:* in a large bowl, stir together the flours, brown sugar, baking powder, cinnamon, bicarbonate of soda, and salt until combined. Whisk together the milk and oil.

5 In a separate glass bowl, beat the egg whites until soft white peaks form.

6 Now, pour the milk and oil mixture into the dry ingredients, and mix with a rubber spatula until moist. Fold in the egg whites gently.  Do not overmix.

7 Scoop the muffin mixture evenly into the paper cases and sprinkle with the crumb topping. Gently press the crumb topping into batter.

8 Bake for 15–17 minutes, or until a toothpick inserted into the centre comes out clean.

9 Turn the muffins out onto a wire rack and allow to cool for at least 10–15 minutes before serving.

| NUTRITION PER SERVING | | | |
|---|---|---|---|
| ENERGY | 1,381kJ (329kcal) | FAT | 10.1g |
| CARBOHYDRATES | 50g | CHOLESTEROL | 1mg |
| SUGARS | 3g | SODIUM | 277mg |
| DIETARY FIBRE | 2.4g | VITAMIN C | 3% |
| PROTEIN | 6.8g | VITAMIN A | 0% |
| | | IRON | 12% |

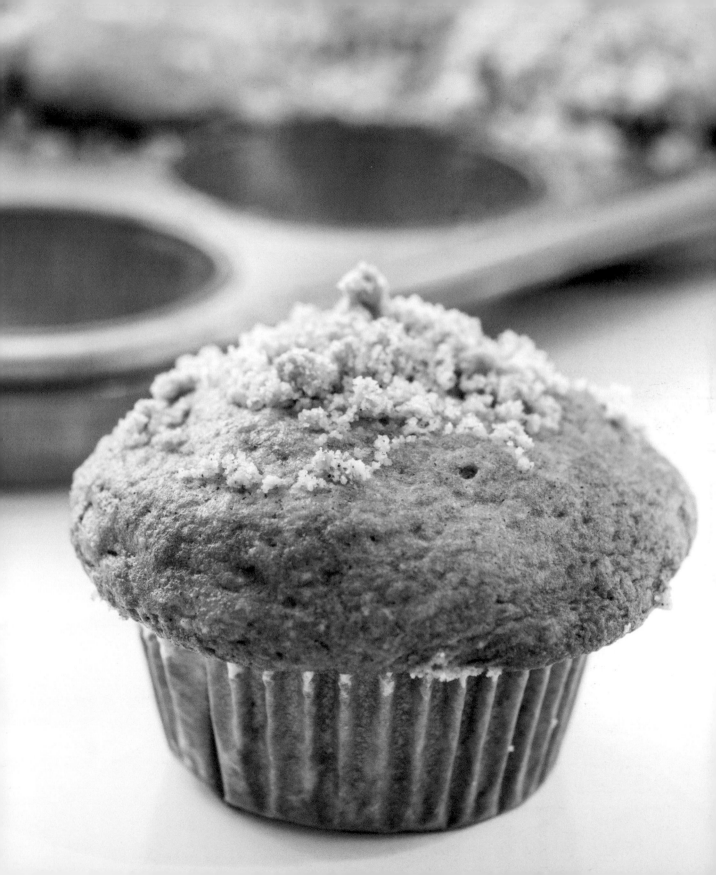

# Raisin Bran **Cookies**

These scrumptious raisin cookies are simple to prepare.
They contain healthy fats and are a source of carbohydrate.

● ● ○ **Intermediate**

**PREP** 10 mins
**COOK** 12–14 mins + cooling

**MAKES** 24

## INGREDIENTS

100g (3½oz) bran flakes
120g (4oz) wholemeal flour
125g (4½oz) plain flour
90g (3oz) granulated sugar
90g (3oz) brown sugar
30g (1oz) pecans, chopped
50g (1¾oz) raisins
½ tsp bicarbonate of soda
4 egg whites
125ml (4fl oz) rapeseed oil
½ tbsp unsweetened apple sauce

1 Preheat the oven to 160°C (325°F/gas 3). Lightly grease a baking tray with cooking spray.

2 In a medium bowl, crush the bran flakes. Add the flours, sugars, pecans, raisins, and bicarbonate of soda, and stir to combine.

3 In a large bowl, beat together the egg whites until soft peaks form.

4 Add the oil and apple sauce to the dry mixture and mix well.

5 Then gradually fold in the egg white into the rest of the mixture.

6 Spoon mounds of cookie dough onto the prepared baking sheet (about 2 tablespoons in size).

7 Bake for 12–14 minutes, or until the cookies are lightly browned. Allow the cookies to cool on a wire rack for 10–12 minutes before storing in an airtight container.

**Make ahead and freeze:** Prepare the cookie dough up to the end of step 7 up to 3 days ahead. You can freeze after step 7 for up to 2 months.

To keep cookies soft, store them with a slice of bread.

| NUTRITION PER SERVING | | | |
|---|---|---|---|
| ENERGY | 596kJ (142kcal) | FAT | 5.7g |
| CARBOHYDRATES | 18.6g | CHOLESTEROL | 0mg |
| SUGARS | 5.7g | SODIUM | 42mg |
| DIETARY FIBRE | 1.7g | VITAMIN C | 0% |
| PROTEIN | 2.4g | VITAMIN A | 6% |
| | | IRON | 8% |

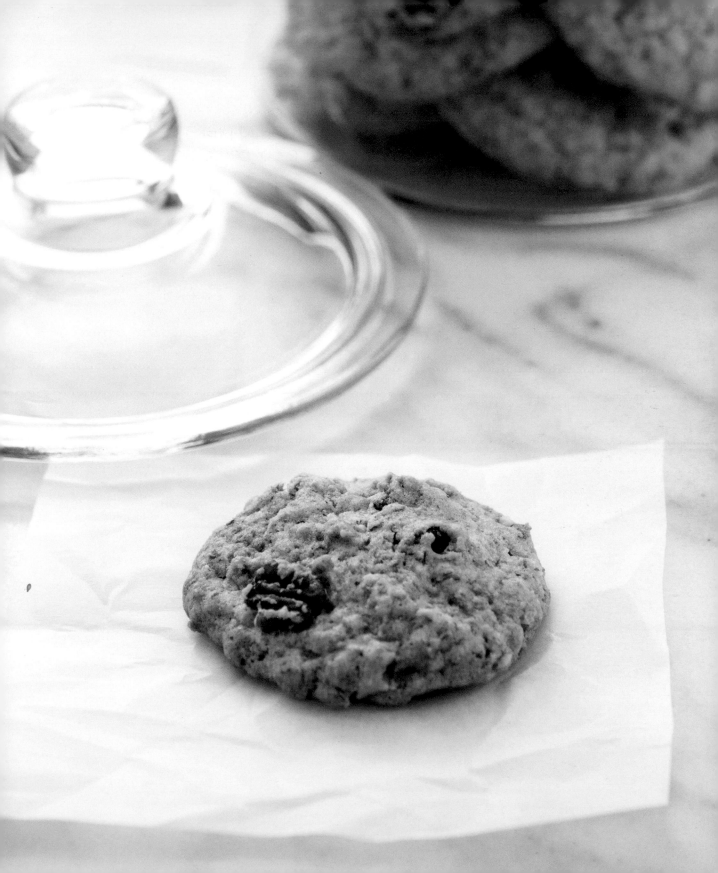

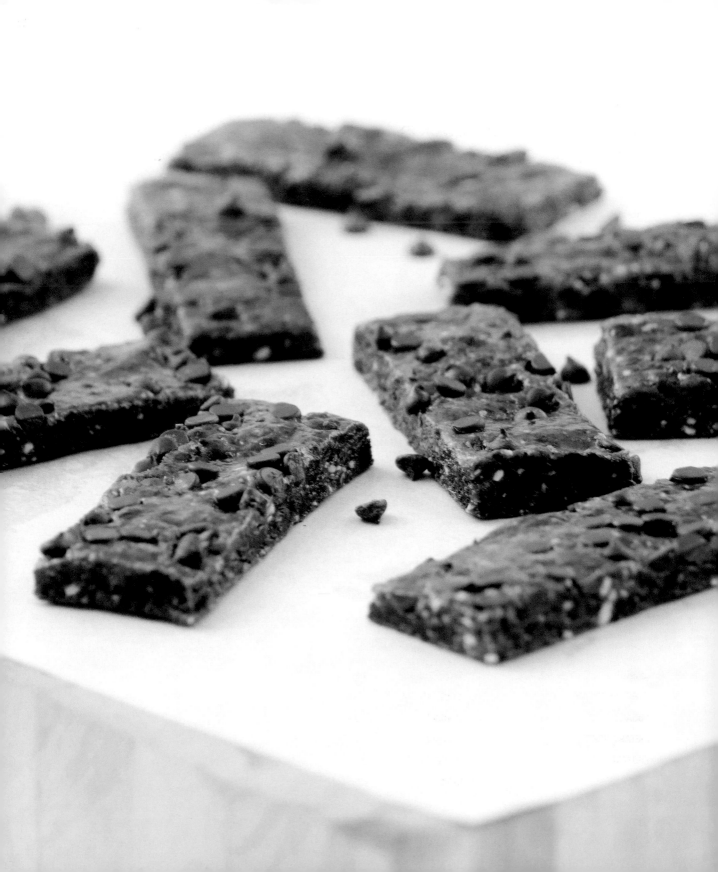

# Quick and Easy **Energy Bars**

These energy bars are quick to make. The recipe is versatile, too: simply mix up the nuts and fruits you use to create your favourite flavour combinations.

**1** Line the bottom of a 20 × 20cm (8 × 8in) baking tray with baking parchment.

**2** In a food processor fitted with a blade, whizz the cashews, cherries, and dates for 25–30 seconds.

**3** Scrape down the sides of the bowl, and whizz again for 1 or 2 minutes or until the ingredients form a ball. Press the mixture evenly into the bottom of the prepared tin.

**4** Sprinkle the chocolate chips over the top, and press into the fruit and nut mixture.

**5** Cover with cling film, and refrigerate overnight.

**6** After the bars have chilled, cut into 8 bars. Wrap each bar individually with cling film, and store in the refrigerator for up to 1 week.

**Make ahead and freeze:** Prepare up to step 6, store in an airtight container at room temperature or refrigerate for up to 1 week, or freeze for up to 1 month.

● **Easy**

**PREP** 10 mins

**MAKES** 8

**INGREDIENTS**

140g (5oz) cashews
160g (5¾oz) dried cherries
150g (5½oz) dried dates
80g (3oz) dark chocolate chips

| NUTRITION PER SERVING | | | |
|---|---|---|---|
| ENERGY | 1,134kJ (270kcal) | FAT | 12g |
| CARBOHYDRATES | 40g | CHOLESTEROL | 0mg |
| SUGARS | 15g | SODIUM | 80mg |
| DIETARY FIBRE | 3g | VITAMIN C | 4% |
| PROTEIN | 4g | VITAMIN A | 8% |
| | | IRON | 6% |

You can enjoy these bars chilled for a firmer bite, or keep them at room temperature if you prefer them a little softer.

# Orange and Ginger **Muffins**

With the sweetness of oranges and the zing of crystallized ginger, these muffins are a tasty treat to have at any time of day – and they also smell fantastic while they're baking! If you prefer a smaller snack, you can divide the mixture into a 12-hole muffin tray.

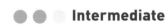 **Intermediate**

**PREP** 10–15 mins
**COOK** 18–20 mins + cooling

**MAKES** 6 large muffins

## INGREDIENTS

125g (4½oz) plain flour
85g (3oz) wholemeal flour
90g (3oz) granulated sugar
1½ tsp baking powder
1½ tsp bicarbonate of soda
½ tsp salt
1 medium orange
30ml (1fl oz) rapeseed oil
1 small ripe banana, mashed
1 large egg
120ml (4fl oz) freshly squeezed
    orange juice
45g (1½oz) crystallized ginger,
    finely chopped

1  Preheat the oven to 190°C (375°F/gas 5). Line a 12-hole muffin tin with paper cases or lightly grease them with cooking spray.

2  In a large bowl, combine the flours, sugar, baking powder, bicarbonate of soda, and salt.

3  Finely zest the orange into a small bowl until you have 1 or 2 tablespoons of zest.

4  Peel and finely chop the orange, removing any seeds, and set aside with the zest.

5  Place the oil and mashed banana in a bowl and whisk them together with an electric whisk on medium speed until combined. Add the egg, then beat until combined.

6  Stir in the chopped orange and orange zest, and gradually whisk in the flour mixture, alternating with orange juice. Fold in the crystallized ginger.

7  Divide the mixture evenly between the cases, and bake for 18–20 minutes, or until a toothpick inserted into centre comes out clean.

8  Turn the muffins out onto a wire rack, and allow to cool for 10–15 minutes. Store leftovers in an airtight container at room temperature, or freeze.

For a tasty flavour variation, add 60g (2oz) dried cranberries when folding in the crystallized ginger.

| NUTRITION PER SERVING | | | |
|---|---|---|---|
| ENERGY | 1,175kJ (280kcal) | FAT | 6.1g |
| CARBOHYDRATES | 47g | CHOLESTEROL | 35mg |
| SUGARS | 21g | SODIUM | 195mg |
| DIETARY FIBRE | 3.5g | VITAMIN C | 35% |
| PROTEIN | 5.3g | VITAMIN A | 1% |
| | | IRON | 9% |

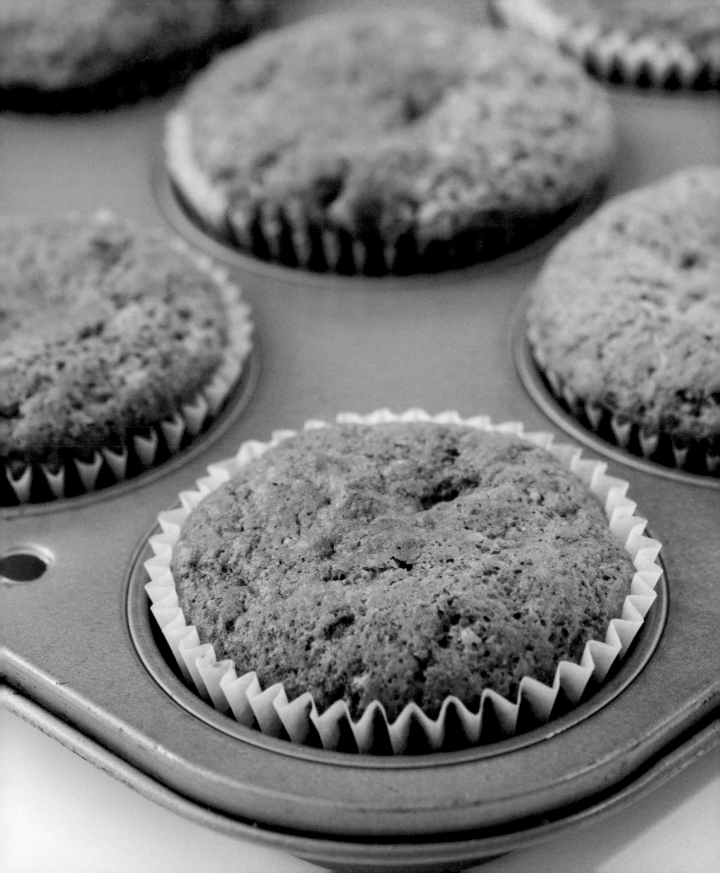

# Bean and Vegetable **Soup**

This hearty and satisfying soup is full of flavour, and is a good source of carbs and protein, especially for the cooler months. Avoid eating close to training, as pulses can cause gastro-intestinal discomfort such as bloating and flatulence.

● ◌ ◌ ◌     **Easy**

**PREP** 10 mins
**COOK** about 3 hours

**SERVES** 8

## INGREDIENTS

2 tbsp extra-virgin olive oil

1 medium sweet yellow
   onion, chopped

120ml (4fl oz) dry white wine
   (optional)

270g (9½oz) dried mixed beans,
   soaked in water overnight
   and drained

1 litre (1¾ pints) low-sodium
   chicken stock

2 litres (3½ pints) low-sodium
   beef stock

3 bay leaves

800g (1¾lb) canned whole
   tomatoes, crushed by hand

2 tbsp chopped fresh parsley

2 tsp chopped fresh thyme

1 tsp chopped fresh oregano

160g (5¾oz) uncooked wild rice

720g (1lb 9oz) frozen mixed
   vegetables

½ tsp salt

¼ tsp freshly ground
   black pepper

1  In a large pan over a medium–high heat, heat the olive oil. Add the onion and cook, stirring occasionally, for 10–15 minutes or until it becomes a deep golden-brown colour.

2  Add the white wine and deglaze, stirring to remove any browned bits from the bottom of the pan. Cook for 2–3 minutes or until the liquid is almost completely absorbed.

3  Add the mixed beans, stocks, and bay leaves. Bring to the boil, cover, reduce the heat to medium, and simmer for about 2 hours or until the beans are almost tender. Skim off and discard any scum from the surface during cooking.

4  Stir in the tomatoes, parsley, thyme, oregano, and wild rice, and simmer for about 20 30 minutes or until the rice and beans are tender.

5  Stir in the mixed vegetables, and cook for about 10 minutes or until cooked through. Season the soup with salt and black pepper, and remove the bay leaves.

6  Serve immediately and freeze portions for use later.

**Make ahead and freeze:** Prepare up to the end of step 5 up to 6 days ahead. Freeze in individual containers after step 5 for up to 2 months.

| NUTRITION PER SERVING | | | |
|---|---|---|---|
| ENERGY | 1,512kJ (360kcal) | FAT | 6g |
| CARBOHYDRATES | 54g | CHOLESTEROL | 0mg |
| SUGARS | 10g | SODIUM | 420mg |
| DIETARY FIBRE | 6g | VITAMIN C | 25% |
| PROTEIN | 19g | VITAMIN A | 25% |
| | | IRON | 25% |

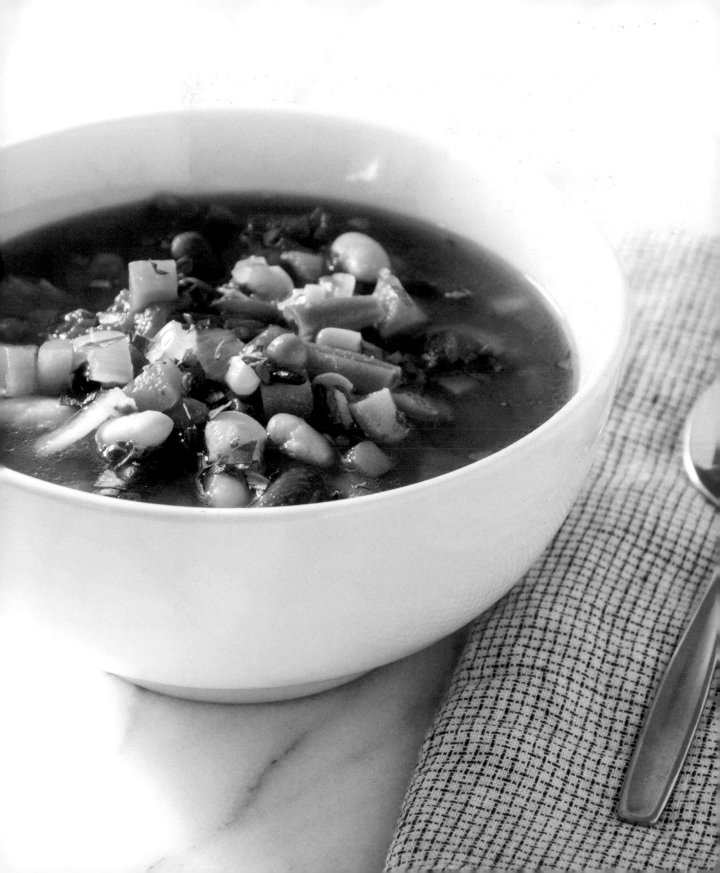

# Lentil **Soup**

This is a brothy soup for a cold day. It is perfect to eat right away, or to prepare in a large batch and freeze in individual servings for later. Legumes can cause gastro intestinal discomfort during training.

● ● ●    **Easy**

**PREP** 10 mins
**COOK** 1 hour

**SERVES** 10

## INGREDIENTS

3 litres (5¼ pints) low-sodium
    chicken or vegetable stock

350g (12oz) dried lentils, rinsed

2 tbsp extra-virgin olive oil

1 large yellow onion, chopped

3 large carrots, peeled
    and chopped

2 tsp balsamic vinegar

½ tsp salt

½ tsp freshly ground
    black pepper

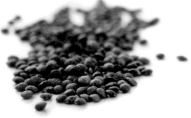

Try a Moroccan spin on this recipe by substituting red lentils, and adding a 410g (14½oz) tin of tomatoes and 2tsp each of cumin, ground coriander, turmeric and cinnamon.

**1** In a large pan over a high heat, heat the stock with the lentils. Bring to the boil, reduce the temperature to low, and simmer for about 1 hour or until the lentils are tender. Skim off and discard any scum from the surface of the soup during cooking.

**2** Meanwhile, heat the oil in a large frying pan over a medium heat. Add the onion, and cook for about 5 minutes or until softened.

**3** Add the carrots, and cook for about 5 minutes or until slightly tender. Remove from the heat, and set aside.

**4** During the last 15–20 minutes of lentil cooking time, add the onions and carrots to the lentils. Stir in the balsamic vinegar, salt, and pepper, and continue to cook.

**5** Serve hot.

**Make ahead and freeze:** Prepare up to the end of step 4 up to 6 days ahead. Freeze in individual containers after step 4 for up to 2 months.

| NUTRITION PER SERVING | | | |
|---|---|---|---|
| ENERGY | 1,008kJ (240kcal) | FAT | 4g |
| CARBOHYDRATES | 37g | CHOLESTEROL | 0mg |
| SUGARS | 3g | SODIUM | 220mg |
| DIETARY FIBRE | 9g | VITAMIN C | 4% |
| PROTEIN | 15g | VITAMIN A | 70% |
| | | IRON | 20% |

# Vegetable and Crab **Soup**

Fuel up for your workout with this delicious Maryland-style crab soup with vegetables. Crab is a lean protein source and this soup is a good source of vitamins A and C.

1 In a large pan over a medium–high heat, combine all of the ingredients except the crabmeat. Bring to the boil, reduce the heat to medium, and simmer, covered, for 5–10 minutes.

2 Stir in the crabmeat, cover, and simmer for 10–15 minutes more.

3 Serve immediately.

**Make ahead and freeze:** Prepare up to the end of step 2 up to 6 days ahead. Freeze in individual containers after step 2 for up to 2 months.

 **Easy**

**PREP** 5 mins
**COOK** about 25 mins

**SERVES** 10

**INGREDIENTS**

2 x 400g (14oz) tins chopped
  tomatoes, with juice
720ml (1¼ pints) water
550g (1¼lb) frozen mixed
  vegetables
1 small sweet yellow onion, diced
2 tbsp Creole Seasoning
480ml (15½fl oz) low-sodium
  beef stock
450g (1lb) white or
  brown crabmeat

| NUTRITION PER SERVING | | | |
|---|---|---|---|
| ENERGY | 504kJ (120kcal) | FAT | 1g |
| CARBOHYDRATES | 11g | CHOLESTEROL | 55mg |
| SUGARS | 5g | SODIUM | 450mg |
| DIETARY FIBRE | 2g | VITAMIN C | 25% |
| PROTEIN | 13g | VITAMIN A | 25% |
| | | IRON | 6% |

If you don't eat seafood, replace crabmeat with cooked chicken.

# Classic Chef **Salad**

This quick, high-protein salad can be easily carried in a cooler bag. For extra carboydrate, add tinned chickpeas or whole kernel sweetcorn.

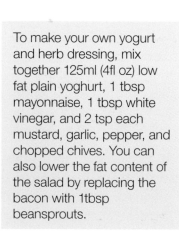

● ○ ○ **Easy**

**PREP** 10 mins

**SERVE** 2

## INGREDIENTS

2 large handfuls of mixed salad leaves

75g (2½oz) ham, sliced

40g (1½oz) turkey, sliced

1 small red onion, sliced

75g (2½oz) cherry tomatoes

40g (1½oz) mozzarella cheese, sliced

30g (1oz) reduced-fat Cheddar cheese, sliced

2 large hard-boiled eggs, peeled and cut in quarters

15g (½oz) bacon bits

70ml (2¼fl oz) yogurt and herb dressing

To make your own yogurt and herb dressing, mix together 125ml (4fl oz) low fat plain yoghurt, 1 tbsp mayonnaise, 1 tbsp white vinegar, and 2 tsp each mustard, garlic, pepper, and chopped chives. You can also lower the fat content of the salad by replacing the bacon with 1tbsp beansprouts.

1 Evenly divide the mixed salad greens between two bowls or large plates. Top with the ham, turkey, red onion slices, cherry tomatoes, mozzarella and Cheddar cheeses, hard-boiled eggs, and bacon bits.

2 Top with the dressing and enjoy immediately.

**Make ahead:** Refrigerate the mixed salad leaves, chopped eggs, meats, and vegetables in separate containers for quick assembly.

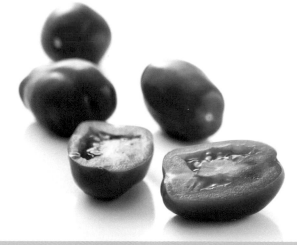

| NUTRITION PER SERVING* | | | |
|---|---|---|---|
| ENERGY | 1,453kJ (346kcal) | FAT | 20.6g |
| CARBOHYDRATES | 7.3g | CHOLESTEROL | 273mg |
| SUGARS | 6.6g | SODIUM | 942mg |
| DIETARY FIBRE | 1.5g | VITAMIN C | 14% |
| PROTEIN | 31.7g | VITAMIN A | 20% |
| | | IRON | 16% |

*Recipe analyzed without dressing included.

# Chickpea **Salad**

This simple marinated salad is so flavoursome and provides a healthy serving of legumes. Make in advance and pack for a portable balanced light lunch or recovery meal.

**1**  Combine all of the ingredients together in a medium bowl.

**2**  Serve chilled or at room temperature.

**Make ahead:** Refrigerate for 3–5 days.

● **Easy**

**PREP** about 10 mins

**SERVES** 2

### INGREDIENTS

400g (14oz) can chickpeas, drained and rinsed

2 tbsp chopped fresh basil

2 tbsp chopped fresh parsley

2 tbsp fresh lemon juice

2 tsp extra-virgin olive oil

1 garlic clove, chopped finely

30g (1oz) Parmesan cheese, freshly grated

¼ tsp sea salt

¼ tsp freshly ground black pepper

| NUTRITION PER SERVING | | | |
|---|---|---|---|
| **ENERGY** | 1,386kJ (330kcal) | **FAT** | 12.8g |
| **CARBOHYDRATES** | 28g | **CHOLESTEROL** | 12mg |
| **SUGARS** | 2.5g | **SODIUM** | 491mg |
| **DIETARY FIBRE** | 8.5g | **VITAMIN C** | 36% |
| **PROTEIN** | 18g | **VITAMIN A** | 13.5% |
| | | **IRON** | 33.5% |

You can transform this recipe into a tasty hummus. In a food processor, blend the chickpeas, lemon juice, oil, garlic, Parmesan, salt, and pepper along with 2 tablespoons tahini paste for 3–5 minutes, or until smooth. Top with the chopped basil and parsley, and serve with pittas or vegetable crudités.

# Easy Italian **Pasta Salad**

This light pasta salad has a refreshing crunch with fresh peppers and onions; it also makes a super side dish for any meal. If you're sensitive to raw onions or peppers, swap them for an alternative.

● ○ ○ **Easy**

**PREP** 10 mins + 1–2 hours marinating
**COOK** about 8 mins

**SERVES** 8

## INGREDIENTS

350g (12oz) tri-coloured fusilli
500g (1lb 2oz) chicken strips
½ medium green pepper, deseeded and diced
½ medium red pepper, deseeded and diced
½ medium red onion, diced
30ml (1fl oz) Italian salad dressing
90g (3oz) sliced black olives, drained
180g (6oz) small fresh mozzarella balls, drained
40g (1¼oz) Italian seasoning
50g (1¾ oz) Parmesan cheese, freshly grated

1 Bring a large pan of water to the boil over a medium–high heat, and cook the pasta for about 8 minutes or until al dente. Drain and rinse the pasta with cold water until cool.

2 In a large bowl, combine the cooled, cooked pasta with the rest of the ingredients and mix gently to combine.

3 Refrigerate for at least 1–2 hours before serving.

**Make ahead:** Refrigerate for 3–5 days.

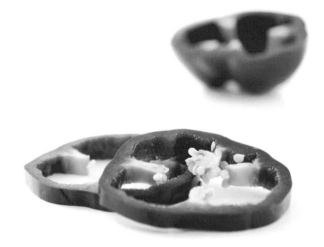

| NUTRITION PER SERVING | | | |
|---|---|---|---|
| ENERGY | 1,512kJ (360kcal) | FAT | 13g |
| CARBOHYDRATES | 31.4g | CHOLESTEROL | 53mg |
| SUGARS | 1.8g | SODIUM | 325mg |
| DIETARY FIBRE | 2.4g | VITAMIN C | 19% |
| PROTEIN | 27g | VITAMIN A | 13% |
| | | IRON | 11% |

# Slow Cooker **Pot Roast**

This dish is a great winter warmer that is easy to prepare. Prepare it in the morning and it will be ready in time for dinner. Serve with rice or quinoa and some extra vegetables to make a complete meal.

1 Use a 5.5-litre (9½-pint) or larger slow cooker. Brown the meat in the oil in a deep frying pan, remove and place in the slow cooker.

2 Fry the onions and garlic in the same pan, and add the spices. Cook for 1 minute on medium heat. Add the remaining ingredients, stir, and transfer to the slow cooker.

3 Cover and cook on high for 3–4 hours or on low for 8–9 hours, whichever suits you best.

4 Stir, and serve immediately.

**Storage:** Refrigerate leftovers for 3–5 days.

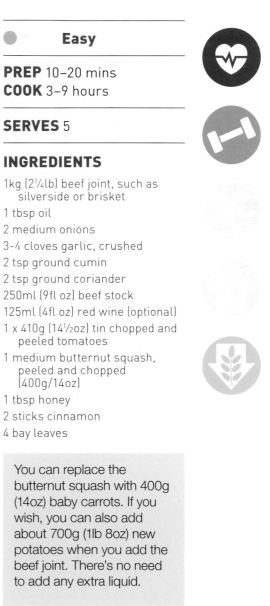

● **Easy**

**PREP** 10–20 mins
**COOK** 3–9 hours

**SERVES** 5

## INGREDIENTS

1kg (2¼lb) beef joint, such as silverside or brisket
1 tbsp oil
2 medium onions
3-4 cloves garlic, crushed
2 tsp ground cumin
2 tsp ground coriander
250ml (9fl oz) beef stock
125ml (4fl oz) red wine (optional)
1 x 410g (14½oz) tin chopped and peeled tomatoes
1 medium butternut squash, peeled and chopped (400g/14oz)
1 tbsp honey
2 sticks cinnamon
4 bay leaves

You can replace the butternut squash with 400g (14oz) baby carrots. If you wish, you can also add about 700g (1lb 8oz) new potatoes when you add the beef joint. There's no need to add any extra liquid.

## NUTRITION PER SERVING

| | | | |
|---|---|---|---|
| ENERGY | 1,747kJ (416kcal) | FAT | 15.6g |
| CARBOHYDRATES | 12.6g | CHOLESTEROL | 116mg |
| SUGARS | 6.6g | SODIUM | 363mg |
| DIETARY FIBRE | 3g | VITAMIN C | 14% |
| PROTEIN | 42.8g | VITAMIN A | 18% |
| | | IRON | 39% |

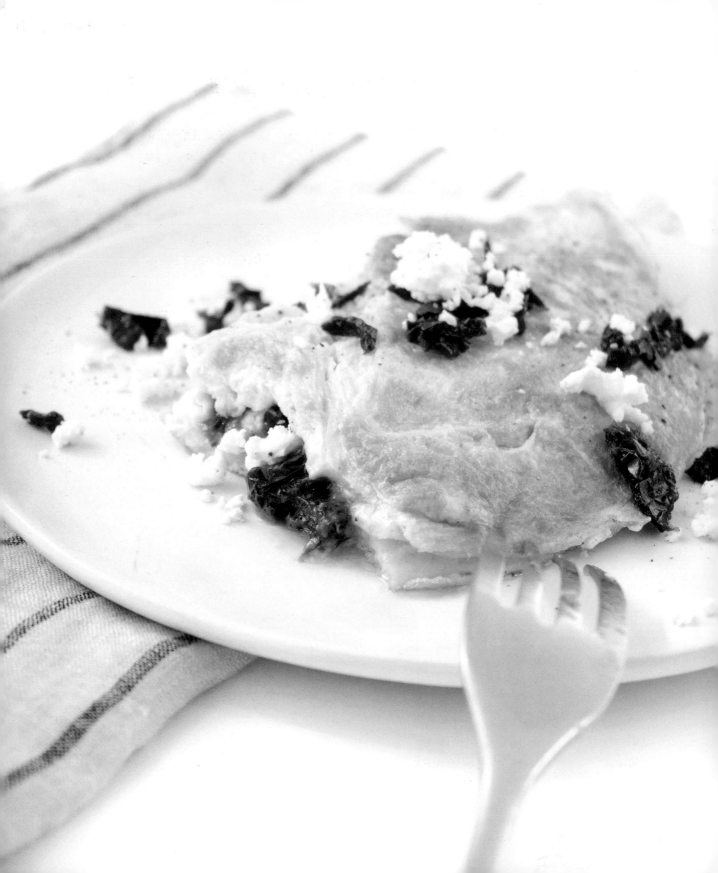

# Sun-Dried Tomato and Feta **Omelette**

Give your body an ample helping of protein with this super tasty omelette. Serve with bread, fresh fruit, and salad for a balanced meal.

**1** Heat the oil in a small frying pan over a medium heat. Add the eggs and cook, swirling eggs with a fork as they set, for 1–2 minutes.

**2** When the eggs are still slightly runny in the middle, scatter sun-dried tomatoes and feta cheese over the top, and fold the omelette in half. Season with black pepper.

**3** Cook for a further minute before sliding the omelette onto a plate and serving.

● **Easy**

**PREP** 5 mins
**COOK** about 3 mins

**SERVES** 1

**INGREDIENTS**

1 tsp extra-virgin olive oil

2 large eggs, lightly beaten

4 sun-dried tomatoes, roughly chopped

2 tbsp crumbled feta cheese

1/8 tsp freshly ground black pepper

## NUTRITION PER SERVING

| ENERGY | 1,092kJ (260kcal) | FAT | 16g |
|---|---|---|---|
| CARBOHYDRATES | 11g | CHOLESTEROL | 435mg |
| SUGARS | 5g | SODIUM | 650mg |
| DIETARY FIBRE | 2g | VITAMIN C | 8% |
| PROTEIN | 18g | VITAMIN A | 20% |
| | | IRON | 15% |

To lower the fat content, use reduced fat feta cheese. To boost protein intake, add 60g (2oz) lean ham.

# Wholemeal and Oat **Pancakes**

These wholegrain flavoursome pancakes are healthier than classic homemade ones. If you like, serve them with blueberries and honey for additional carbohydrate.

● ○ ○ **Easy**

**PREP** 5 mins
**COOK** 5–10 mins for
all pancakes

**SERVES** 3

**INGREDIENTS**

75g (2½oz) quick-cooking oats
360ml (12fl oz) plus 2 tbsp
buttermilk
90g (3¼oz) wholemeal flour
1½ tsp baking powder
¾ tsp bicarbonate of soda
½ tsp ground cinnamon
⅛ tsp grated nutmeg
1 large egg, lightly beaten
1 tbsp vegetable oil
1½ tbsp brown sugar
blueberries and honey to
serve (optional)

1 In a medium bowl, combine the oats and 180ml (6fl oz) of buttermilk. Set aside to soak for about 10 minutes.

2 Meanwhile, heat a griddle pan over a medium heat. Lightly grease with cooking spray.

3 In a large bowl, stir together the wholemeal flour, baking powder, bicarbonate of soda, cinnamon, and nutmeg.

4 Stir in the egg, oil, and brown sugar, remaining buttermilk and the oat–buttermilk mixture, until just combined.

5 Pour about 4 tablespoons of batter (or 60ml/2fl oz) per pancake onto the hot griddle, and cook for about 1 minute or until bubbles appear on the surface of the pancake and the underneath is golden brown. Flip the pancake with a spatula, and cook the other side for about 30 seconds to 1 minute.

6 Serve immediately with blueberries and honey, if desired.

**Storage:** You can freeze leftover pancakes, defrost them, and reheat them under a hot grill to serve.

Swap blueberries and honey for maple syrup and bananas, apple or pear slices, or strawberries. Reduce the fibre content by using white flour instead of wholemeal.

| NUTRITION PER SERVING | | | |
|---|---|---|---|
| ENERGY | 1,407kJ (335kcal) | FAT | 9g |
| CARBOHYDRATES | 52g | CHOLESTEROL | 80mg |
| SUGARS | 14g | SODIUM | 760mg |
| DIETARY FIBRE | 6g | VITAMIN C | 2% |
| PROTEIN | 14g | VITAMIN A | 4% |
| | | IRON | 15% |

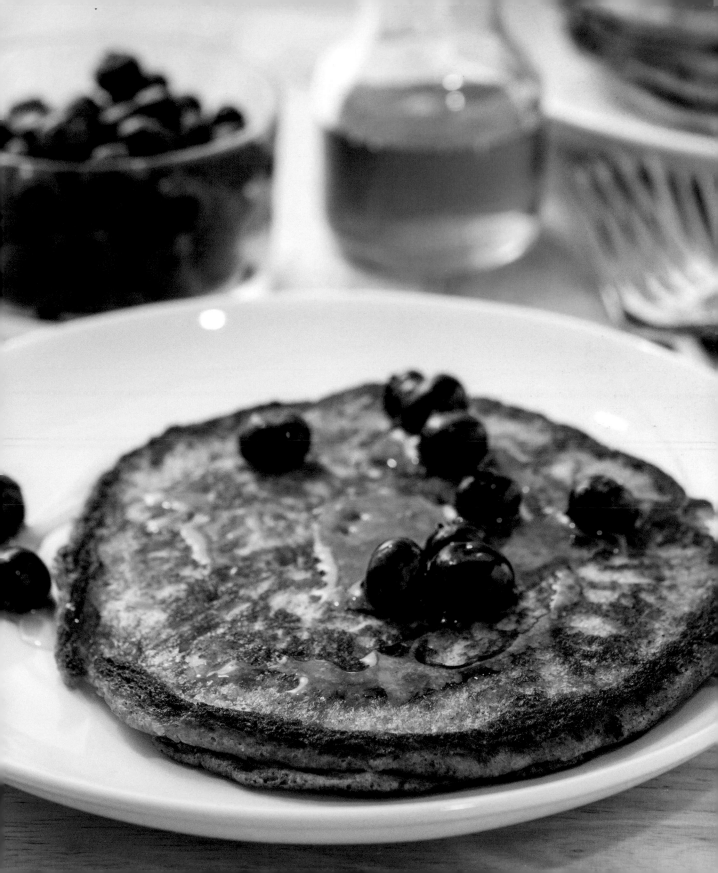

# Stuffed Courgette **Boats**

This dish is high in protein and a good source of iron. Serve with a wholegrain bread roll to bulk up carbohydrate intake. Aubergines can be used instead of courgettes.

● ● ○ **Intermediate**

**PREP** 10–15 mins
**COOK** 40–50 mins

**SERVES** 8

## INGREDIENTS

4 large courgettes

1 tbsp extra-virgin olive oil

500g (1lb 2oz) extra-lean mince

1 small red onion, finely chopped

450g (1lb) cherry tomatoes, halved

1 tsp sea salt

½ tsp freshly ground black pepper

40g (1½oz) panko breadcrumbs

25g (scant 1oz) Parmesan cheese, freshly grated

2 tbsp chopped fresh parsley or 1 tbsp dried parsley

For a vegetarian alternative, you could substitute a drained and rinsed 400g (14oz) tin of chickpeas for the mince. Cook the chickpeas, red onion, and tomatoes together until the tomatoes start to break down. Continue with the recipe as above.

1   Preheat the oven to 180°C (350°F/gas 4). Lightly grease a baking tray with cooking spray.

2   Place a large, deep frying pan over a medium–high heat. Add the courgettes, cover halfway with water, and bring to a simmer. Reduce the heat to low, cover, and cook for 6–8 minutes or until tender-crisp. Remove from the heat.

3   Drain and dry the frying pan. Set over a medium-high heat, and add extra-virgin olive oil and extra-lean mince. Cook, stirring, for about 4 minutes. Stir in the red onion, and cook for about 4 minutes. Add cherry tomatoes, season with salt and pepper, and cook for 1 minute, or until the tomatoes start to cook down. Remove from the heat.

4   Slice the courgettes in half lengthways. Scoop out the centres, making a boat shape. Chop the scooped-out flesh and add to the mince mixture. Divide the mince between the courgette shells, and set the courgettes on the baking tray.

5   In a small bowl, combine the breadcrumbs, Parmesan cheese, and parsley. Sprinkle over the stuffed courgettes.

6   Bake for about 25 minutes, or until the topping is golden brown and the courgettes are cooked through. Serve hot.

| NUTRITION PER SERVING | | | |
|---|---|---|---|
| ENERGY | 1,428kJ (340kcal) | FAT | 13.2g |
| CARBOHYDRATES | 14.6g | CHOLESTEROL | 94mg |
| SUGARS | 7g | SODIUM | 758mg |
| DIETARY FIBRE | 4.1g | VITAMIN C | 61% |
| PROTEIN | 36.8g | VITAMIN A | 12% |
| | | IRON | 37% |

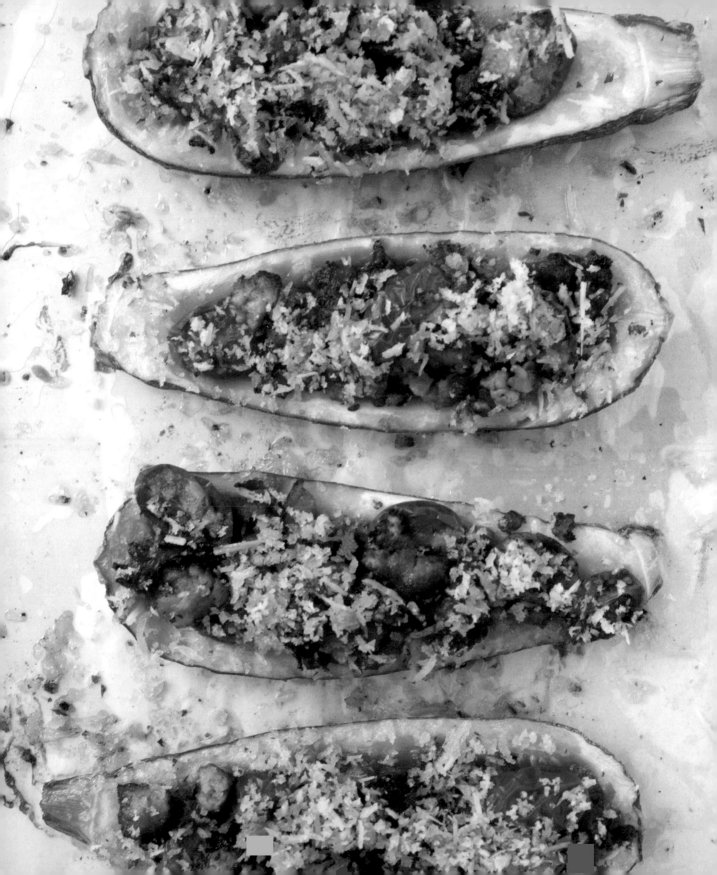

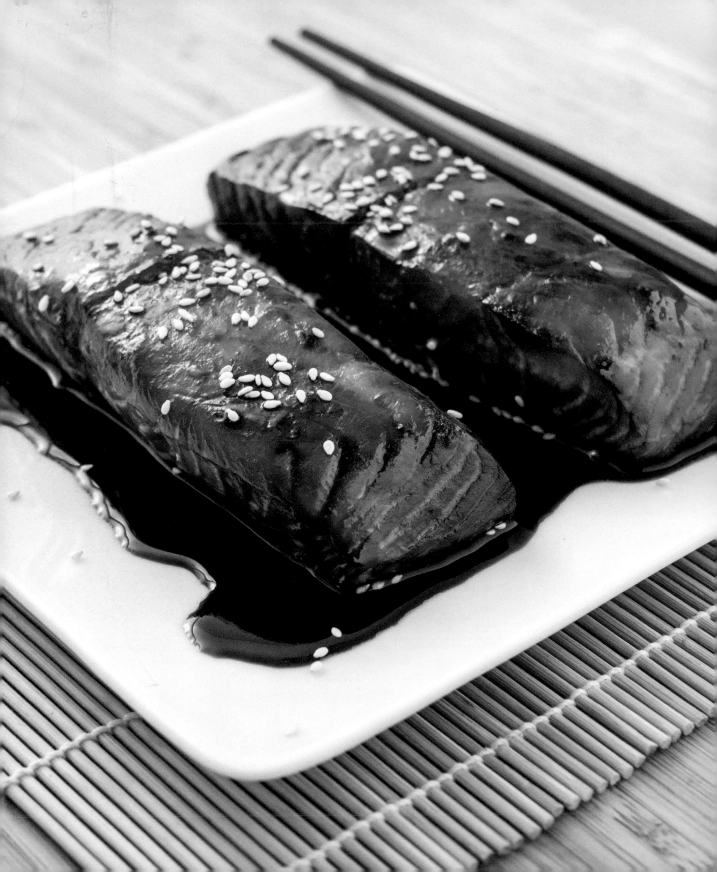

# **Teriyaki** Salmon

Pair this sticky and sweet dish with stir-fried vegetables, or serve over an Asian-inspired salad. Salmon is a good source of omega 3.

1 In a small pan over a low heat, combine the sesame oil, orange juice, soy sauce, sugar, sesame seeds, mustard, ginger, black pepper, and garlic powder. Bring to a simmer, stirring until all the sugar has dissolved. Set aside 120ml (4fl oz) of this marinade.

2 Pour the remaining marinade into a zip-lock plastic bag with the salmon steaks, and marinate in the refrigerator for 1–2 hours.

3 Preheat the grill and set the shelf about 10cm (4in) from the heat.

4 Remove the salmon steaks, discarding the marinade, and place them on a baking sheet. Place the sheet under the grill, and cook for 5 minutes.

5 Brush the salmon with half the reserved marinade, turn over, and grill for a further 5 minutes or until the salmon is cooked through.

6 Remove the salmon from the heat, flip over the steaks, top with the remaining marinade, and cover with foil. Allow the fish to rest, covered, for 5–10 minutes before serving.

**Make ahead and freeze:** Prepare up to the end of step 2 up to 3 days ahead. Freeze after step 2 for up to 2 months.

**Easy**

**PREP** 10 mins + 1–2 hours marinating
**COOK** 20 mins

**SERVES** 4

**INGREDIENTS**

1 tbsp sesame oil
Juice of 1 medium orange
4 tbsp low-sodium soy sauce
2 tbsp brown sugar, packed
1 tbsp sesame seeds
1 tsp mustard powder
1 tsp ground ginger
¼ tsp freshly ground black pepper
¼ tsp garlic powder
4 x 115g (4oz) salmon steaks

| NUTRITION PER SERVING | | | |
|---|---|---|---|
| ENERGY | 1,306kJ (311kcal) | FAT | 19g |
| CARBOHYDRATES | 10g | CHOLESTEROL | 60mg |
| SUGARS | 8g | SODIUM | 460mg |
| DIETARY FIBRE | 0g | VITAMIN C | 8% |
| PROTEIN | 25g | VITAMIN A | 2% |
| | | IRON | 4% |

# Chickpea and Cauliflower **Tacos**

This vegetarian dish is rich in carbohydrate and protein. Cauliflower is also known for its antioxidant properties, and is high in vitamin C.

● ● ○ **Intermediate**

**PREP** 2 mins
**COOK** 1 hour, 5 mins

**SERVES** 4

## INGREDIENTS

1 medium cauliflower, separated into florets (about (1kg/2¼lb)
3 tbsp extra-virgin olive oil
1 tsp sea salt
400g (14oz) tin chickpeas, drained and rinsed
¼ tsp chilli powder
¼ tsp ground cumin
¼ tsp dried oregano
120ml (4fl oz) salsa verde
8 x 15cm (6in) corn tortillas

1 Preheat the oven to 220°C (425°F/gas 7).

2 Put the cauliflower florets in a large bowl. Drizzle with 2 tablespoons of the extra-virgin olive oil, sprinkle with ½ teaspoon of the salt, and stir until evenly coated.

3 Arrange the florets on a large baking tray and bake for 15 minutes. Stir the cauliflower and bake for a further 15–20 minutes or until the cauliflower is browned.

4 Meanwhile, in a small bowl, combine the chickpeas, chilli powder, cumin, oregano, and remaining salt.

5 Spread the chickpea mixture into a 23 × 33cm (9 × 13in) baking tin, and bake for 15 minutes. Stir the chickpeas, and bake for a further 10–15 minutes, or until the chickpeas are slightly browned and crispy.

6 Spoon about 1 tablespoon of salsa verde onto each corn tortilla, and top with about 8 tablespoons of roasted cauliflower and 1 tablespoon of crisp chickpeas.

7 Serve immediately.

**Storage:** Refrigerate leftover filling for 3–5 days.

Make your own salsa verde by blending 100ml (3½oz) olive oil, 1 anchovy fillet, 1 garlic clove, and 2 tbsp capers with parsley and mint. Add red wine vinegar, salt and pepper to taste.

| NUTRITION PER SERVING | | | | |
|---|---|---|---|---|
| EMERGY | 1,397kJ (333kcal) | | FAT | 15g |
| CARBOHYDRATES | 56g | | CHOLESTEROL | 0mg |
| SUGARS | 9g | | SODIUM | 960mg |
| DIETARY FIBRE | 11g | | VITAMIN C | 190% |
| PROTEIN | 11g | | VITAMIN A | 4% |
| | | | IRON | 15% |

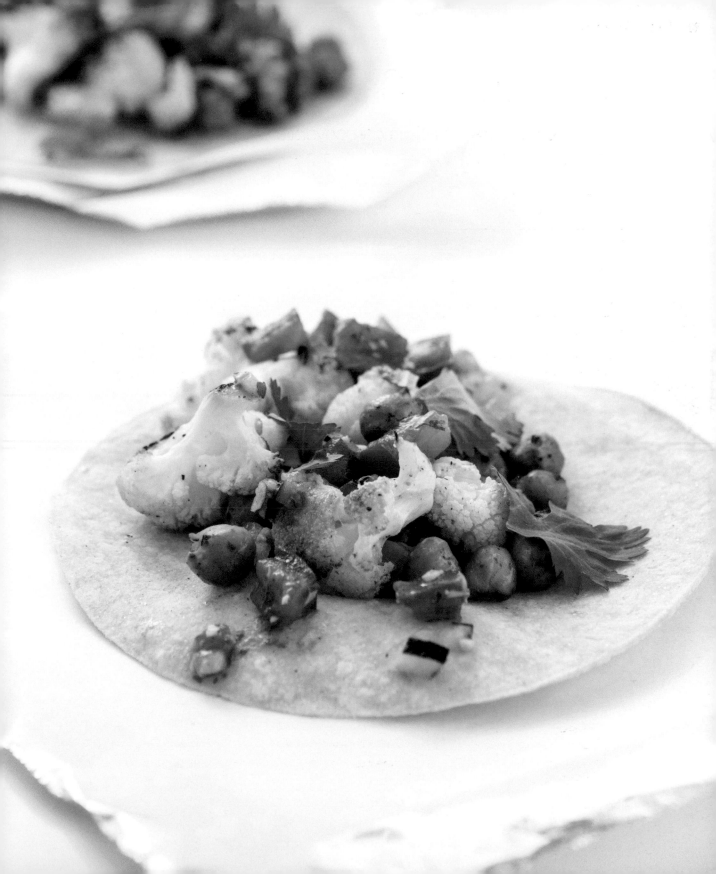

# Three Cheese and Spinach
# **Stuffed Shells**

An excellent dish for the whole family, these stuffed shells feature fresh wilted spinach, garlic, and three kinds of cheese. They are good source of protein, carbohydrate, iron, and vitamins A and C.

● ● ● **Intermediate**

**PREP** 10 mins
**COOK** 40 mins

**SERVES** 8

## INGREDIENTS

24 jumbo pasta shells
    (about 225g/8oz)

1½ tsp extra-virgin olive oil

2 small sweet yellow
    onions, chopped

900g (2lb) fresh baby
    spinach, washed

500g (1lb 2oz) low-fat
    ricotta cheese

40g (1¼oz) fresh breadcrumbs

50g (1¾oz) Parmesan
    cheese, grated

125g (4½oz) low-fat
    mozzarella cheese

¼ tsp ground nutmeg

¼ tsp garlic salt

1 tsp salt

½ tsp freshly ground
    black pepper

1 large egg white, lightly beaten

720ml (1¼ pints) ready-made
    tomato pasta sauce

1  Preheat the oven to 190°C (375°F/gas 5).

2  Cook the pasta shells in a large pan of boiling water over a medium–high heat, stirring often, for about 15 minutes. Drain, rinse under cool water, and set aside.

3  Heat the oil in a large frying pan over a medium–high heat. Add the onions and cook, stirring occasionally, for about 3 minutes, or until softened.

4  Add the baby spinach in batches, and toss until wilted. Drain the spinach in a colander and press out the excess liquid. Set aside.

5  In a large bowl, combine the ricotta cheese, breadcrumbs, half of the Parmesan, mozzarella, and nutmeg. Add the spinach, onion, garlic salt, salt, and black pepper, and stir in the egg white. Stuff each pasta shell with 2 tablespoons of this cheese mixture.

6  Spread 240ml (8fl oz) of the tomato sauce on the bottom of a 23 × 33cm (9 × 13in) baking dish. Add the stuffed shells in a single layer, top with remaining tomato sauce, and sprinkle with the remaining Parmesan. Bake for about 30 minutes. Cool for 5–10 minutes before serving.

| NUTRITION PER SERVING | | | |
|---|---|---|---|
| ENERGY | 1,470kJ (350kcal) | FAT | 6g |
| CARBOHYDRATES | 55g | CHOLESTEROL | 15mg |
| SUGARS | 5g | SODIUM | 1,210mg |
| DIETARY FIBRE | 9g | VITAMIN C | 30% |
| PROTEIN | 21g | VITAMIN A | 90% |
| | | IRON | 30% |

# Prawn and Spinach **Pasta**

This vibrant dish combines fresh spinach and succulent prawns with the flavours of lemon, basil, and Parmesan cheese. Prawns are a lean source of protein, and are rich in B vitamins, zinc, selenium and omega-3 fatty acids.

1 In a large pan over a medium–high heat, cook the pasta according to the packet instructions. Ladle 240ml (8fl oz) of pasta water into a small bowl, and set aside. Drain the pasta, return to the pan, cover, and set aside.

2 Meanwhile, heat the oil in a large frying pan over a medium–high heat. Add the prawns and garlic, and cook, stirring occasionally, for about 2 minutes.

3 Add the tomatoes with juice, half the basil, the lemon juice, and lemon zest, and sauté for about 3 minutes or until the prawns are cooked through.

4 Add the baby spinach to the hot pasta, and toss until the spinach wilts. Add the prawn mixture, and toss to combine. Add the reserved pasta water, and stir in the Parmesan, salt, black pepper, and the remaining basil.

5 Serve immediately.

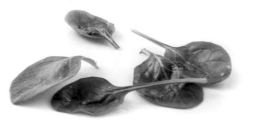

● **Easy**

**PREP** 10 mins
**COOK** about 15 mins

**SERVES** 4

## INGREDIENTS

350g (12 oz) tri-colored fusilli pasta

1 tbsp extra-virgin olive oil

450g (1lb) raw prawns, peeled and deveined

3 cloves garlic, finely chopped

400g (14oz) tin chopped tomatoes, with juice

15g (½oz) fresh basil, chopped

3 tbsp fresh lemon juice

2 tsp lemon zest

225g (8oz) fresh baby spinach, washed

25g (scant 1oz) Parmesan cheese, grated

1 tsp salt

½ tsp freshly ground black pepper

To make this recipe vegetarian, use 400g (14oz) of tinned chickpeas, drained and rinsed, instead of the prawns.

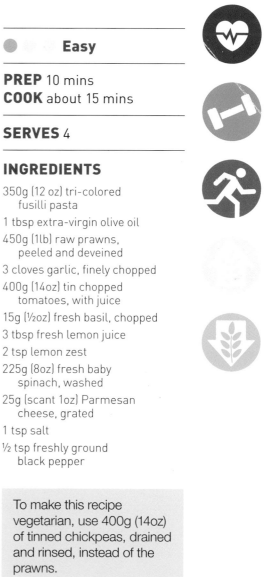

### NUTRITION PER SERVING

| ENERGY | 2,117kJ (504kcal) | FAT | 7g |
|---|---|---|---|
| CARBOHYDRATES | 76g | CHOLESTEROL | 175mg |
| SUGARS | 6g | SODIUM | 1,240mg |
| DIETARY FIBRE | 6g | VITAMIN C | 60% |
| PROTEIN | 39g | VITAMIN A | 60% |
| | | IRON | 35% |

# Beef, Broccoli, and Sweet Potato **Stir-Fry**

This super stir-fry is loaded with lean protein and carbohydrates. Sweet potatoes are an are an excellent source of vitamin A, an antioxidant that is key to a healthy immune system and good vision.

● **Easy**

**PREP** 15 mins
**COOK** about 10 mins

**SERVES** 4

## INGREDIENTS

60ml (2fl oz) water

1 tbsp brown sugar

3 tbsp oyster sauce

450g (1lb) beef skirt, cut into 5mm x 1.25cm (¼ × ½in) slices

½ tsp salt

½ tsp freshly ground black pepper

1½ tbsp cornflour

1 tbsp sesame oil

250g (9oz) broccoli florets

1 sweet potato (225g (8oz)), cut into 7.5mm (⅓in) slices

2 tsp fresh root ginger, peeled and finely chopped

¼ tsp crushed chilli flakes

Feel free to use different protein sources in this recipe, such as chicken or prawn. If you cannot find oyster sauce, substitute with soy sauce.

1 In small bowl, combine the water, brown sugar, and oyster sauce until the sugar has dissolved. Set the sauce aside.

2 Place the beef in a large bowl. Sprinkle with the salt, black pepper, and cornflour, and toss to coat.

3 In a wok or a large frying pan over a high heat, heat 1½ tablespoons of the sesame oil. Add the coated beef, and stir-fry for about 3 minutes or until the beef is no longer pink outside. Transfer the beef to a medium bowl.

4 Return the frying pan to the heat, and add the remaining sesame oil. Toss in the broccoli florets, sweet potato slices, and root ginger, and toss to coat.

5 Sprinkle the crushed chilli flakes into the frying pan along with the reserved sauce. Cover, reduce the heat to medium–high, and cook for about 5 minutes or until the vegetables are just tender.

6 Return the beef to the frying pan, and toss to coat it for about 1 minute. Serve hot.

**Storage:** Refrigerate leftovers for 3–5 days.

| NUTRITION PER SERVING | | | |
|---|---|---|---|
| ENERGY | 1,285kJ (306kcal) | FAT | 13g |
| CARBOHYDRATES | 16g | CHOLESTEROL | 60mg |
| SUGARS | 4g | SODIUM | 740mg |
| DIETARY FIBRE | 5g | VITAMIN C | 70% |
| PROTEIN | 33g | VITAMIN A | 2% |
| | | IRON | 15% |

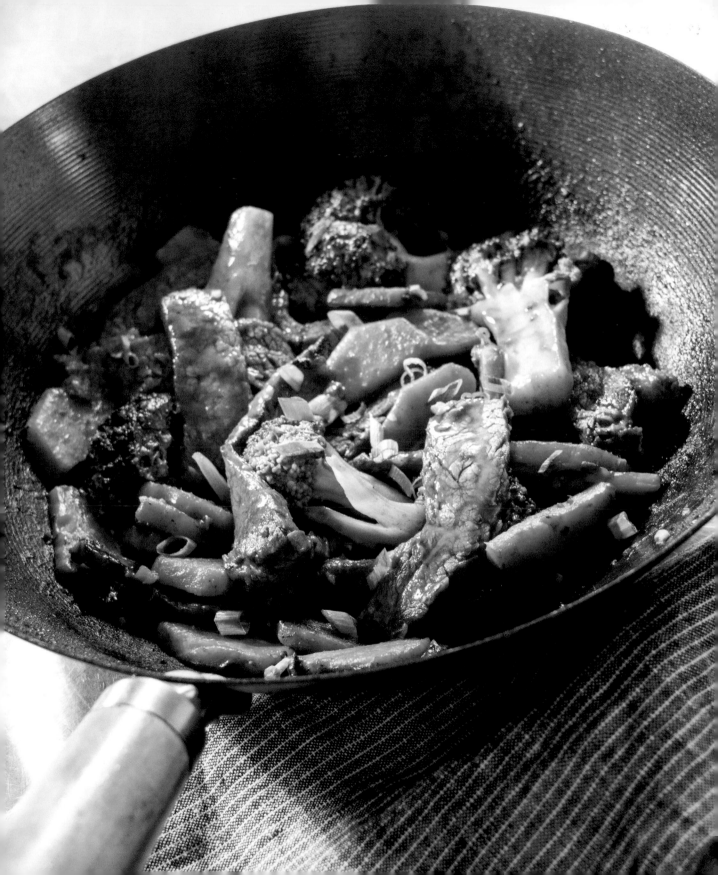

# Simple Chicken **Marsala**

This simple chicken dish, with fresh mushrooms and sweet Marsala wine, is both quick to prepare and satisfying. Serve with rice and lightly steamed vegetables for a complete meal.

● ● ◯ **Intermediate**

**PREP** 5–10 mins
**COOK** about 16 mins

**SERVES** 4

## INGREDIENTS

30g (1oz) plain flour

½ tsp garlic salt

¼ tsp freshly ground black pepper

1 tsp fresh oregano

4 x 115g (4oz) boneless, skinless chicken breasts

2 tbsp extra-virgin olive oil

85g (3oz) button mushrooms, sliced

120ml (4fl oz) Marsala wine

1 In a medium bowl, combine the flour, garlic salt, black pepper, and oregano.

2 Dredge both sides of the chicken breasts in the seasoned flour until lightly coated. Set aside.

3 Heat the oil in a large frying pan over a medium heat. Add the chicken to the pan, and sear for 2–3 minutes or until lightly browned on one side.

4 Turn over the chicken, add the mushrooms, and cook for a further 2–3 minutes or until the other side of the chicken is lightly browned as well. Stir the mushrooms occasionally to ensure they cook evenly.

5 Pour the Marsala wine over the chicken, cover the pan, reduce the heat to low, and simmer for 10 minutes or until the chicken is cooked through.

6 Serve hot immediately.

**Storage:** Refrigerate leftovers for 3–5 days.

To make this recipe gluten free, choose a gluten-free plain flour instead.

| NUTRITION PER SERVING | | | |
|---|---|---|---|
| ENERGY | 868kJ (207kcal) | FAT | 9g |
| CARBOHYDRATES | 10g | CHOLESTEROL | 55mg |
| SUGARS | 3g | SODIUM | 220mg |
| DIETARY FIBRE | 0g | VITAMIN C | 2% |
| PROTEIN | 19g | VITAMIN A | 0% |
| | | IRON | 4% |

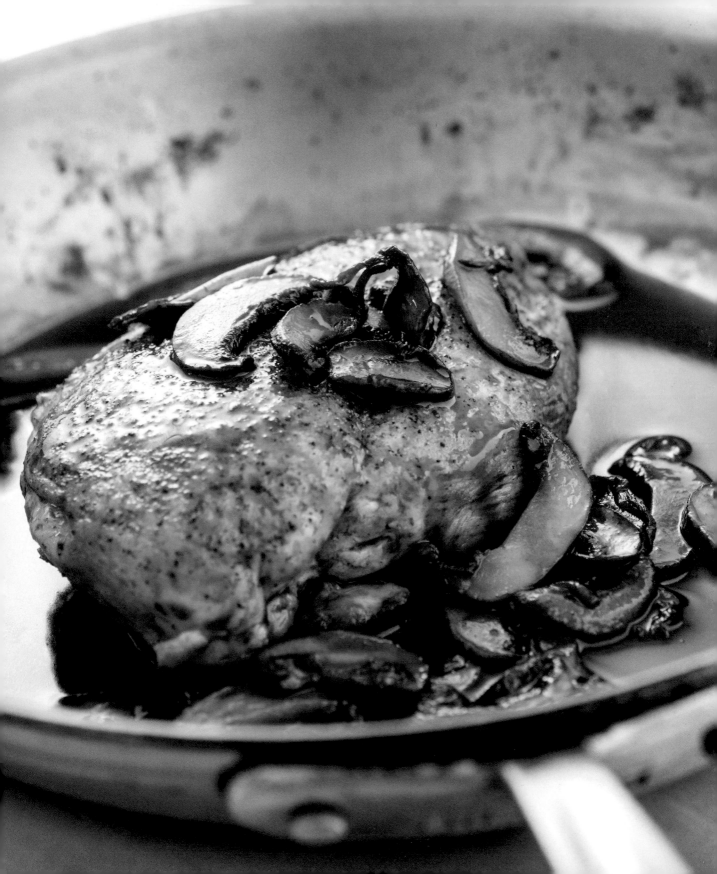

# Slow Cooker **Rice Pudding**

This old-fashioned rice pudding is packed full of carbs to keep your body energized. It's perfect year round: served warm for winter sports or chilled during summer events.

● ○ ○    **Easy**

**PREP** 5 mins
**COOK** 2½–3 hours

**SERVES** 6

## INGREDIENTS

140g (5oz) long-grain white rice
80g (2¾oz) raisins
720ml (1¼ pints)
    semi-skimmed milk
120g (4oz) granulated sugar
1 tsp ground cinnamon
½ tsp salt
30g (1oz) unsalted butter, melted

1  Lightly grease a 4-litre (7-pint) slow cooker with cooking spray.

2  In a colander, rinse the long-grain white rice thoroughly under cold water.

3  Transfer the rice to the slow cooker. Add the raisins, milk, sugar, cinnamon, and salt, and stir to combine.

4  Pour the melted butter over the rice mixture and stir to combine. Cover, and cook on high for 2½–3 hours or until the rice has absorbed all the liquid.

5  Serve warm or chilled.

**Storage:** Refrigerate leftovers for 3–5 days.

To add more carbohydrate to this recipe, stir in 120g (4¼oz) sultanas, dried cherries, or chopped dried apricots when you add the butter.

### NUTRITION PER SERVING

| | | | | |
|---|---|---|---|---|
| ENERGY | 1,277kJ (304kcal) | FAT | 6.8g |
| CARBOHYDRATES | 53g | CHOLESTEROL | 19mg |
| SUGARS | 35g | SODIUM | 189mg |
| DIETARY FIBRE | 1g | VITAMIN C | 1% |
| PROTEIN | 6g | VITAMIN A | 8% |
| | | IRON | 3.5% |

# Strawberry and Yogurt **Ice Lollies**

This wonderful summery treat is perfect for keeping cool and providing carbohydrate for before or after your workout. It also makes a brilliant treat for children, instead of regular ice cream.

**1** In a medium bowl, combine the strawberries, agave syrup, and vanilla extract. Set aside for 15–20 minutes.

**2** In a blender, purée the strawberry mixture along with the low-fat plain yogurt until smooth.

**3** Evenly divide the mixture between 6 ice lolly moulds, and freeze for about 4 hours or until firm.

**Storage:** Keep frozen for up to 2–3 months.

● **Easy**

**PREP** 20 mins + 4 hours freezing

**MAKES** 6

**INGREDIENTS**

325g (11oz) fresh strawberries, hulled and sliced

3 tbsp agave syrup or honey

2 tsp vanilla extract

240ml (8fl oz) low fat plain yogurt

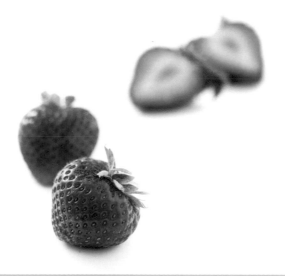

| NUTRITION PER SERVING | | | |
|---|---|---|---|
| ENERGY | 563kJ (134kcal) | FAT | 1g |
| CARBOHYDRATES | 28g | CHOLESTEROL | 3mg |
| SUGARS | 6g | SODIUM | 30mg |
| DIETARY FIBRE | 1g | VITAMIN C | 40% |
| PROTEIN | 2.2g | VITAMIN A | 0% |
| | | IRON | 4% |

If sugar isn't your preferred sweetener, you can use 4 tablespoons of agave nectar or honey instead.

# Blueberry Orange **Parfaits**

Whip up these tasty parfaits, made with fresh blueberries and sweet oranges. Packed with carbohydrate, protein, calcium, and vitamin C, these can make an appetising breakfast or a healthy dessert.

● ● ● **Easy**

**PREP** 15 mins

**SERVES** 4

## INGREDIENTS

½ tsp orange zest (from the oranges below)

480ml (15½fl oz) low-fat plain yogurt

300g (10oz) fresh blueberries

2 large oranges, broken into segments

125g (4½oz) granola cereal

1 In a small bowl, combine the orange zest and low-fat plain yogurt.

2 Spoon about one-eighth of the blueberries into 4 parfait or tall glasses, followed by about 2½ tablespoons yogurt mixture and one-eighth of the orange segments each. Repeat the layers with the remaining blueberries, yogurt mixture, and orange segments.

3 Sprinkle each serving with one-quarter of the granola.

4 Serve immediately.

**Make ahead:** Refrigerate the prepared fruit and yogurt for quick assembly.

If you cannot find blueberries, substitute for strawberries and lime juice, or banana and passion fruit.

| NUTRITION PER SERVING | | | |
|---|---|---|---|
| ENERGY | 1,399kJ (333kcal) | FAT | 7.5g |
| CARBOHYDRATES | 49g | CHOLESTEROL | 17mg |
| SUGARS | 34g | SODIUM | 119mg |
| DIETARY FIBRE | 8.7g | VITAMIN C | 107% |
| PROTEIN | 9g | VITAMIN A | 6% |
| | | IRON | 4% |

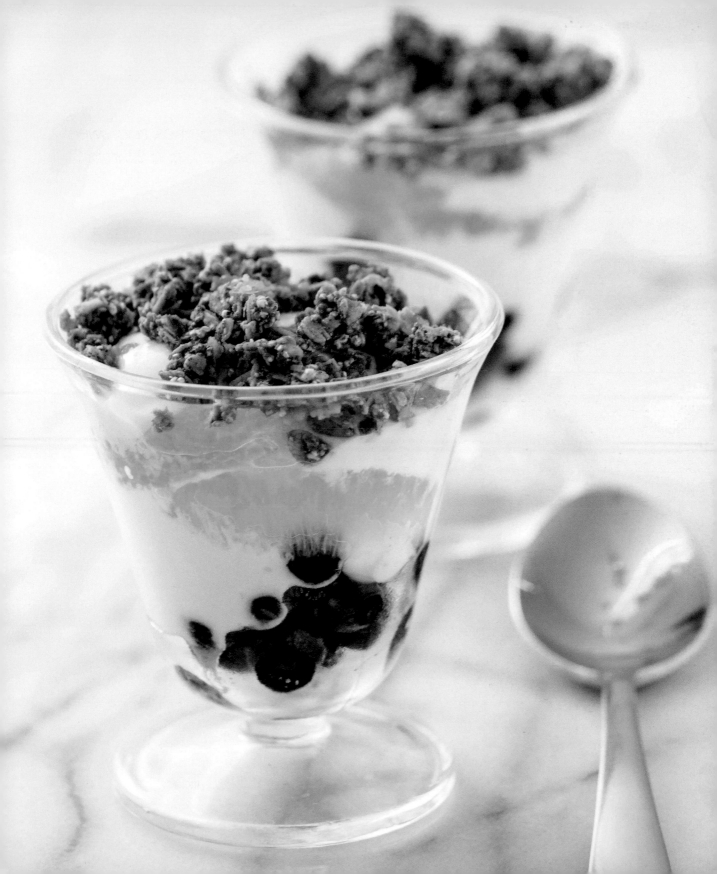

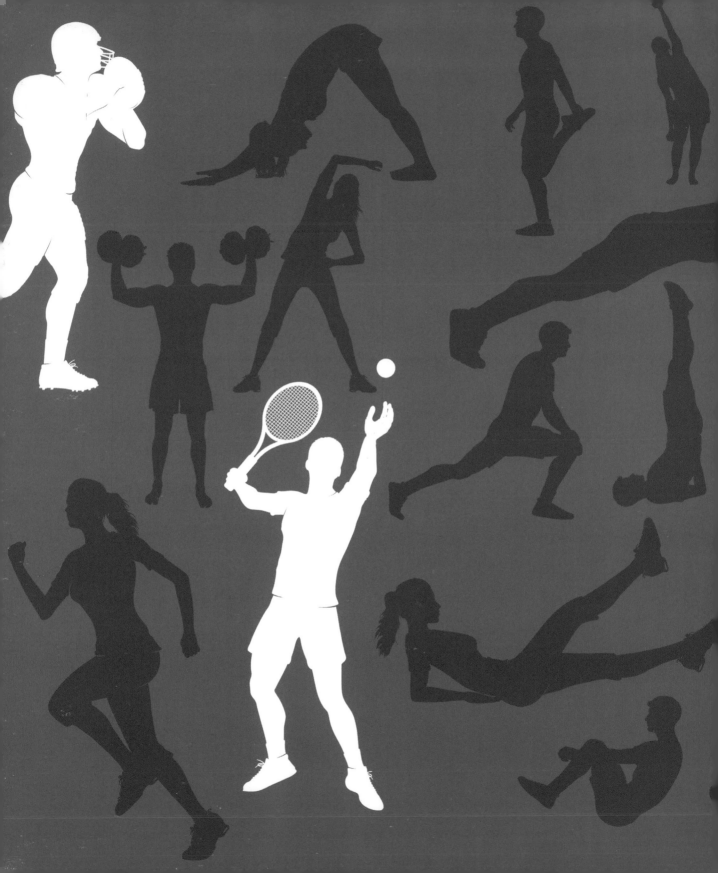

# Recipes for
# **Competition**

Competition meals and snacks
should be high in carbohydrate,
contain a moderate amount of protein
and be low in fat and fibre to avoid
gastrointestinal discomfort.

In Part 3, we give you a number of meals you can take
on the go, including homemade competition sports drinks
and refreshing smoothies - not to mention more delicious
and easy-to-prepare portables.

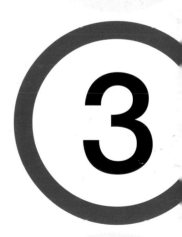

# Mango **Cooler**

Refreshing and delicious, this tropical cooler is just what your body needs to keep you pushing on through your workout. Ideal for quenching your thirst at half time.

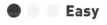 **Easy**

**PREP** 2 mins

**SERVES** 1

## INGREDIENTS

180ml (6fl oz) mango nectar juice

260ml (9fl oz) water

1 tbsp granulated sugar

⅛ tsp salt

1   Combine all the ingredients in a large glass.

2   Drink over ice.

| NUTRITION PER SERVING | | | |
|---|---|---|---|
| **ENERGY** 504kJ (120kcal) | | **FAT** | 0g |
| **CARBOHYDRATES** | 31g | **CHOLESTEROL** | 0mg |
| **SUGARS** | 30g | **SODIUM** | 310mg |
| **DIETARY FIBRE** | 0g | **VITAMIN C** | 15% |
| **PROTEIN** | 0g | **VITAMIN A** | 8% |
| | | **IRON** | 4% |

# Lavendar Lemonade **Relaxer**

This summery lemonade can help boost your carbohydrate intake and calm your nerves during competitions.

● ○ ○  **Easy**

**PREP** 2 hours 10 mins
**COOK** about 5 mins

**SERVES** 1

## INGREDIENTS

65g (2¼ oz) granulated sugar

80ml (2½fl oz) water

2 tbsp dried lavender flowers

120ml (4fl oz) lemon juice

240ml (8fl oz) cold water

⅛ tsp salt

1   In small pan over a medium–high heat, bring the sugar and water to the boil. Add the lavender flowers, remove from the heat, and set aside for 2 hours. Strain the syrup and discard the lavender.

2   Stir in the lemon juice, water, and salt, and serve over ice.

| NUTRITION PER SERVING | | | |
|---|---|---|---|
| **ENERGY** 798kJ (190kcal) | | **FAT** | 0g |
| **CARBOHYDRATES** | 59g | **CHOLESTEROL** | 0mg |
| **SUGARS** | 51g | **SODIUM** | 300mg |
| **DIETARY FIBRE** | 0g | **VITAMIN C** | 90% |
| **PROTEIN** | 0g | **VITAMIN A** | 0% |
| | | **IRON** | 0% |

Mango Cooler

Lavender Lemonade
Relaxer

# Apple Cinnamon
# **Refresher**

This apple drink is like autumn in a glass, with just a hint of cinnamon. It is lower in sugar than the average sports drink, too.

● ○ ○ **Easy**

**PREP** 5 mins

**SERVES** 3

## INGREDIENTS

Juice of 2 medium oranges
480ml (15½fl oz) water
1½ tsp granulated sugar
750ml (1¼ pints) apple juice
½ tsp ground cinnamon

1  Combine all the ingredients together in a water jug.

2  Consume chilled or over ice.

> Heat to make a warm apple cider drink.

| NUTRITION PER SERVING | | | |
|---|---|---|---|
| ENERGY | 294kJ (70kcal) | FAT | 0g |
| CARBOHYDRATES | 18g | CHOLESTEROL | 0mg |
| SUGARS | 16g | SODIUM | 15mg |
| DIETARY FIBRE | 0g | VITAMIN C | 0% |
| PROTEIN | 0g | VITAMIN A | 0% |
| | | IRON | 0% |

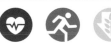

# Pineapple Ginger
# **Sipper**

This carbohydrate rich sipper is sweet due to delicious pineapple juice and a little zesty thanks to the crystallized ginger. Rich in vitamin C.

● ○ ○ **Easy**

**PREP** 3 mins

**YIELD** 1 serving

## INGREDIENTS

420ml (14½fl oz) pineapple juice
120ml (4fl oz) water
1 large piece crystallized ginger, roughly chopped
⅛ tsp salt

1  Combine all the ingredients together in a large glass.

2  Drink over ice.

| NUTRITION PER SERVING | | | |
|---|---|---|---|
| ENERGY | 966kJ (230kcal) | FAT | 0g |
| CARBOHYDRATES | 56g | CHOLESTEROL | 0mg |
| SUGARS | 54g | SODIUM | 300mg |
| DIETARY FIBER | 0g | VITAMIN C | 35% |
| PROTEIN | 0g | VITAMIN A | 4% |
| | | IRON | 4% |

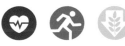

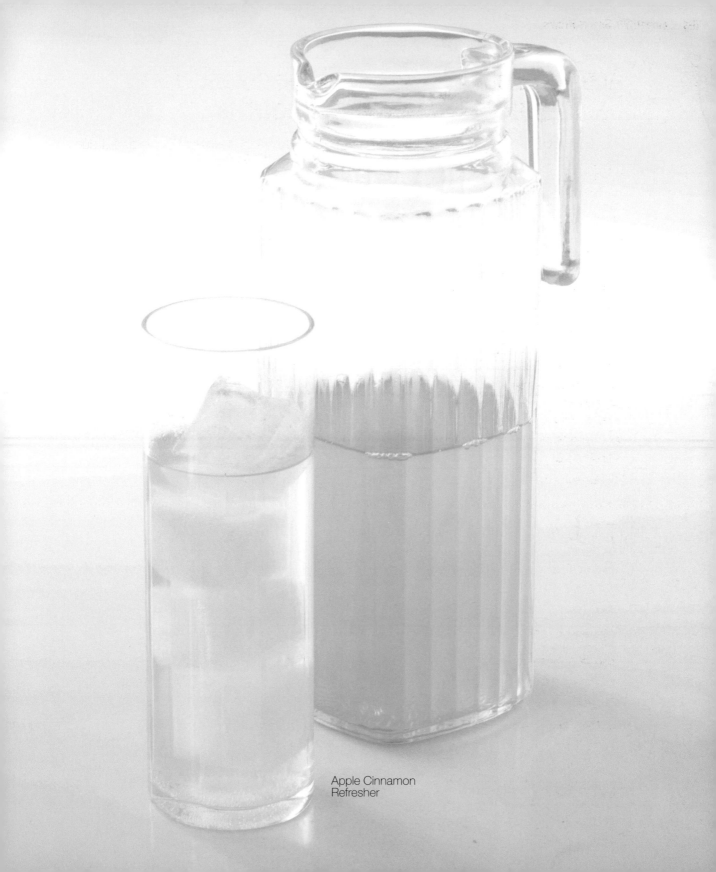

Apple Cinnamon
Refresher

# Creamy Orange and Carrot **Smoothie**

You are sure to love this sweet orange and ginger smoothie full of vitamins and minerals. It provides more than your daily requirement of vitamin C, and a good amount of beta-carotene for eye and skin health.

● ○ ○ **Easy**

**PREP** 3 mins

**SERVES** 1

## INGREDIENTS

75g (2½oz) frozen orange juice concentrate

1 medium carrot, chopped

1 large piece crystallized ginger, roughly chopped

4 tbsp whole milk

180ml (6fl oz) ice cubes

**1** Combine all the ingredients together in a blender for 1–2 minutes, or until smooth.

**2** Drink immediately.

> Use soy milk if you do not tolerate dairy well. Replace whole milk with semi-skimmed to lower the fat content.

| NUTRITION PER SERVING | | | |
|---|---|---|---|
| ENERGY | 798kJ (190kcal) | FAT | 1.5g |
| CARBOHYDRATES | 40g | CHOLESTEROL | 5mg |
| SUGARS | 34g | SODIUM | 110mg |
| DIETARY FIBRE | 3g | VITAMIN C | 140% |
| PROTEIN | 4g | VITAMIN A | 340% |
| | | IRON | 2% |

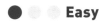

# Lean, Green, Broccoli **Smoothie**

Broccoli is an unexpected ingredient in a smoothie, but this drink is sweet and masks the broccoli flavour well. It is also very high in vitamin C.

● ○ ○ **Easy**

**PREP** 5 mins

**SERVES** 2

## INGREDIENTS

250g (9oz) honeydew or canteloupe melon (weight once peeled and seeded), cubed

360ml (12fl oz) ice cubes

2 kiwis, peeled

½ medium cucumber, peeled, seeded, and chopped

20g (¾oz) fresh broccoli florets

5–10 fresh mint leaves

**1** Combine all the ingredients together in a blender for 2–3 minutes, or until completely combined.

**2** Drink immediately.

| NUTRITION PER SERVING | | | |
|---|---|---|---|
| ENERGY | 882kJ (210kcal) | FAT | 1.5g |
| CARBOHYDRATES | 49g | CHOLESTEROL | 0mg |
| SUGARS | 37g | SODIUM | 60mg |
| DIETARY FIBRE | 8g | VITAMIN C | 360% |
| PROTEIN | 4g | VITAMIN A | 20% |
| | | IRON | 8% |

Creamy Orange and
Carrot Smoothie

Lean, Green,
Broccoli Smoothie

# Country Vegetable **Frittata**

This hearty breakfast dish with vegetables, ham, potato, and Cheddar cheese will get your competition day off to a great start.

● ○ ○ **Easy**

**PREP** 5 mins
**COOK** about 20 mins

**SERVES** 4

## INGREDIENTS

2 tbsp extra-virgin olive oil

handful of baby spinach, diced tomatoes, and peppers (optional)

450g (1lb) cooked potatoes, diced small

30g (1oz) ham, diced

¼ tsp garlic, minced

8 large eggs

1 tsp salt

½ tsp freshly cracked black pepper

30g (1oz) sharp Cheddar cheese, grated

1  Preheat the oven to 180°C (350°F/gas 4).

2  Heat the oil in a 30cm (12in) nonstick frying pan with an ovenproof handle over a medium–high heat. Add the vegetables (if using), potatoes, ham, and garlic, and sauté for about 5 minutes or until lightly browned.

3  In a medium bowl, whisk the eggs with salt and black pepper. Pour the eggs over the potato mixture, reduce the heat to medium–low, and cook, using a rubber spatula to occasionally scrape around the edges of the frittata as it cooks, for 5–10 minutes.

4  When the eggs are nearly set, sprinkle the cheese over the top, and place in the oven for 3–5 minutes or until the eggs are evenly set and slightly golden.

5  Serve hot.

**Storage:** Refrigerate leftovers for 3–5 days.

For a vegetarian version, omit the ham. Vary the vegetables, try peas, baby marrows, or broccoli and feta. For lower fat version, use reduced-fat cheese, or replace or 4 of the eggs with 8 egg whites.

| NUTRITION PER SERVING | | | |
|---|---|---|---|
| ENERGY | 1,235kJ (294kcal) | FAT | 14g |
| CARBOHYDRATES | 25g | CHOLESTEROL | 440mg |
| SUGARS | 1g | SODIUM | 780mg |
| DIETARY FIBRE | 2g | VITAMIN C | 15% |
| PROTEIN | 14g | VITAMIN A | 15% |
| | | IRON | 10% |

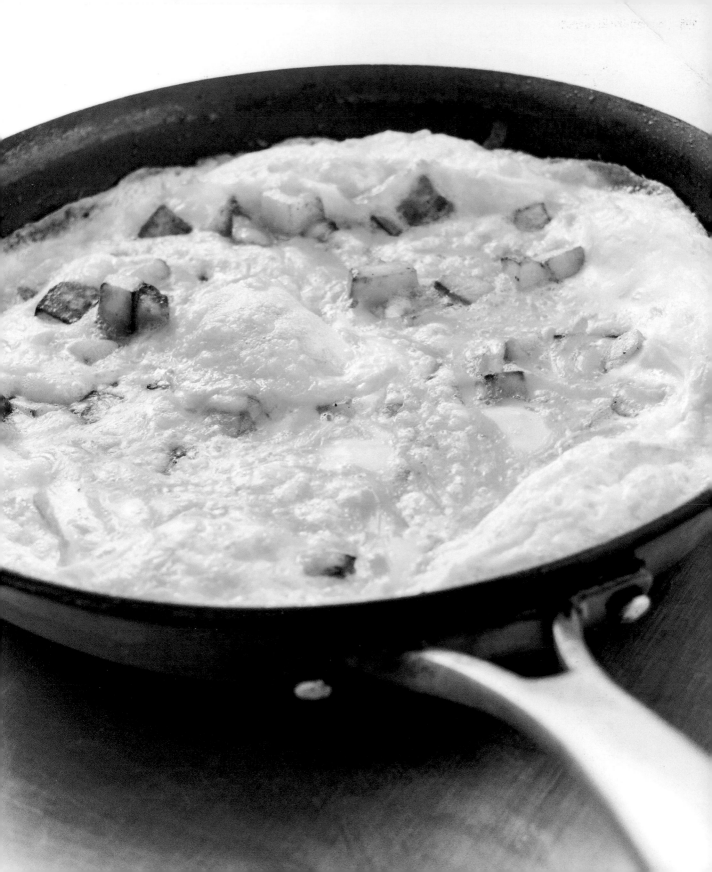

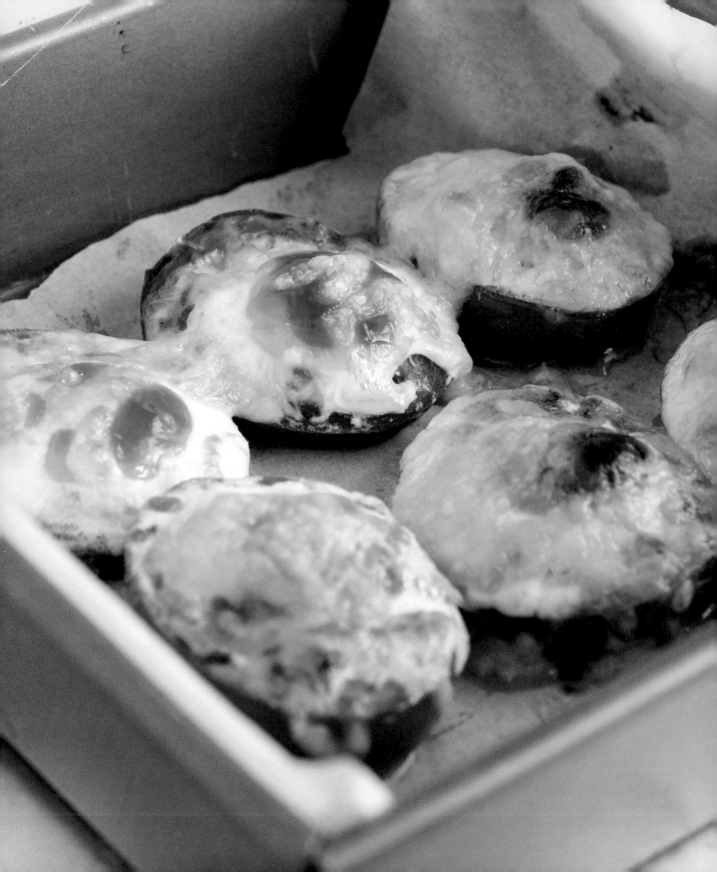

# Baked Egg and Tomato **Cups**

Whether it is for a quick and easy breakfast or an on-the-go treat that gives a good amount of protein, these breakfast cups fit the bill. Serve with a toasted bagel for carbohydrate.

**1** Preheat the oven to 230°C (450°F/gas 8).

**2** Cut the tomatoes in half and remove the seeds. Slice a small sliver off the bottom of each tomato half, so that it stands up steady, and place in a baking tray.

**3** Crack the eggs and gently place 1 egg inside each tomato cup. Season the egg with black pepper, and sprinkle with the mozzarella cheese.

**4** Bake in the oven for 8–10 minutes, or until the eggs are cooked through.

**5** Serve hot, or allow to cool and take on the road chilled.

**Make ahead:** Prepare up to step 4, and refrigerate for up to 5 days.

● ○ ○ **Easy**

**PREP** 8 mins
**COOK** 8–10 mins

**SERVES** 4

**INGREDIENTS**

4 large beefsteak tomatoes

8 small eggs

½ tsp freshly ground black pepper

50g (1¾oz) mozzarella cheese, grated

| NUTRITION PER SERVING | | | |
|---|---|---|---|
| ENERGY | 874kJ (208kcal) | FAT | 12.3g |
| CARBOHYDRATES | 7g | CHOLESTEROL | 387mg |
| SUGARS | 6.8g | SODIUM | 169mg |
| DIETARY FIBRE | 2.2g | VITAMIN C | 45% |
| PROTEIN | 15.5g | VITAMIN A | 20% |
| | | IRON | 16% |

If you can't find beefsteak tomatoes to hold your eggs, use large vine-ripe tomatoes instead.

# Super-Quick Breakfast **Burrito**

Now you no longer have an excuse to skip breakfast on a busy competition day. You can have this super-simple breakfast burrito ready in a matter of minutes.

● ○ ○ **Easy**

**PREP** 2 mins
**COOK** 1 min

**SERVES** 1

## INGREDIENTS

1 x 15cm (6in) wheat tortilla
1 large egg
1 tbsp grated Cheddar cheese
1 tbsp tomato salsa
¼ tsp freshly ground black
   pepper

1  Line a 480ml (15½fl oz) capacity microwave-safe bowl with a sheet of kitchen paper. Press the flour tortilla into the bowl, break the egg into the centre of the tortilla, and beat the egg gently with a fork.

2  Microwave on high power for 30 seconds, stir, and microwave for a further 15–30 seconds or until the egg is almost set.

3  Transfer the tortilla and its kitchen paper liner from the bowl to a flat surface. Top the egg with the cheese, salsa, and black pepper, and roll up the tortilla.

4  Enjoy immediately.

To lower the fat content, use reduced fat cheddar cheese or 2 egg whites instead of the whole egg. If not eating close to a competition, add 2 tbsp black beans and guacamole.

| NU TRITION PER SERVING | | | |
|---|---|---|---|
| ENERGY | 765kJ (180kcal) | FAT | 7g |
| CARBOHYDRATES | 18g | CHOLESTEROL | 215mg |
| SUGARS | 1g | SODIUM | 370mg |
| DIETARY FIBRE | 1g | VITAMIN C | 2% |
| PROTEIN | 10g | VITAMIN A | 8% |
| | | IRON | 10% |

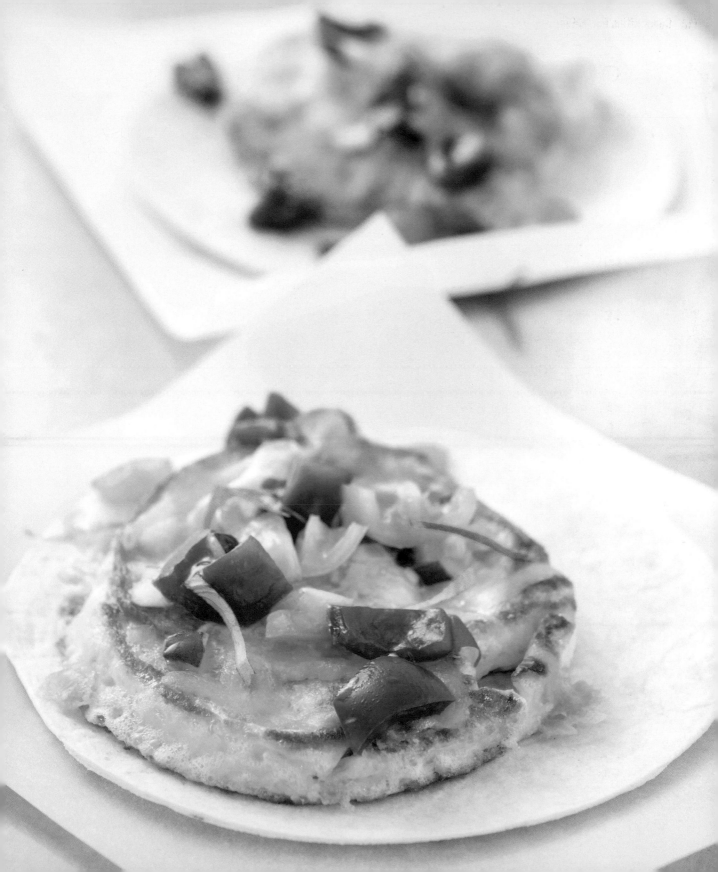

# Low-Fat Banana **Bread**

You will love this update to the classic banana bread recipe – it has the same delicious flavour but is much lower in fat.

● ○ ○ ○ **Easy**

**PREP** 10 mins
**COOK** about 1 hour

**SERVES** 16

## INGREDIENTS

225g (8oz) plain flour, plus extra for dusting

2 large eggs

150g (5½oz) sugar

2 very ripe bananas, peeled and mashed

4 tbsp apple sauce

½ tsp ground cinnamon

80ml (2½fl oz) whole milk

1 tbsp vegetable oil

1 tbsp vanilla extract

2 tsp baking powder

½ tsp bicarbonate of soda

½ tsp salt

40g (1¼ oz) chopped walnuts

1 Preheat the oven to 160°C (325°F/gas 3). Lightly grease 2 x 900g (2lb) loaf tins with cooking spray, dust with flour, and shake out the excess flour.

2 In a large bowl, beat eggs and sugar for about 5 minutes or until light and fluffy.

3 Using a rubber spatula, beat in the bananas, apple sauce, cinnamon, milk, oil, and vanilla extract.

4 In a separate large bowl, sift together the flour, baking powder, bicarbonate of soda, and salt. Stir this dry mixture into the banana mixture, mixing just until blended.

5 Fold in the walnuts, and evenly divide the mixture between the prepared loaf tins.

6 Bake for about 1 hour or until golden and a toothpick inserted into centre of each loaf comes out clean.

7 Turn out the bread onto a wire rack, and allow to cool.

**Make ahead and freeze:** Prepare up to the end of step 5 up to 3 days ahead. Freeze the bread, sliced or whole, at the end of step 7 for up to 2 months.

| NUTRITION PER SERVING | | | |
|---|---|---|---|
| ENERGY | 462kJ (110kcal) | FAT | 3g |
| CARBOHYDRATES | 20g | CHOLESTEROL | 25mg |
| SUGARS | 10g | SODIUM | 190mg |
| DIETARY FIBRE | 0.4g | VITAMIN C | 0% |
| PROTEIN | 3g | VITAMIN A | 0% |
| | | IRON | 4% |

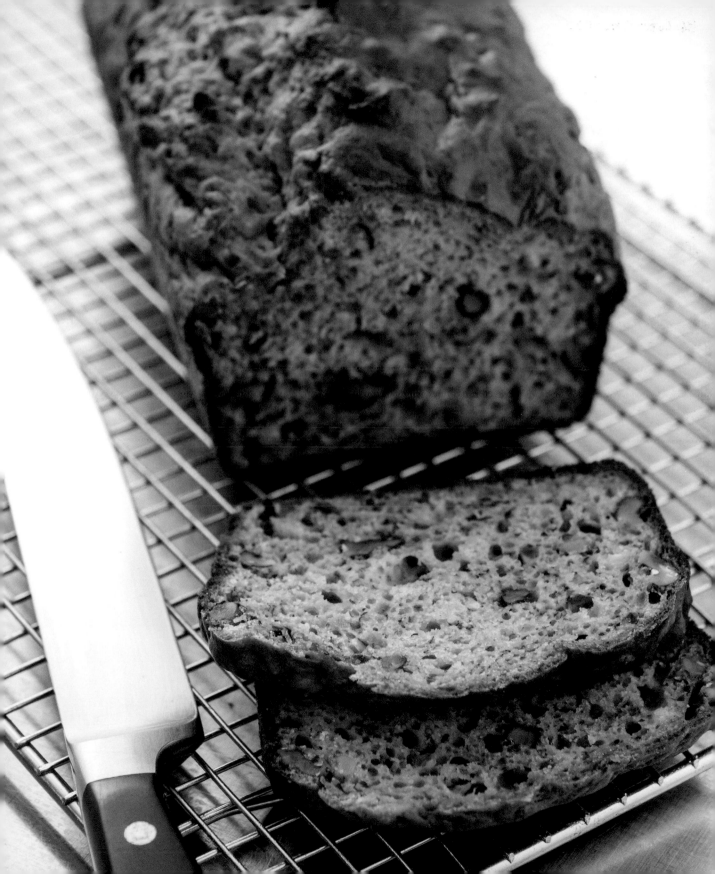

# Turkey and Spring Onion **Wraps**

Wraps are the ultimate form of portable snack – a convenient package of protein and vegetables or salads. Make sure to secure your wrap with foil to prevent the contents spilling out.

● ◌ ◌ **Easy**

**PREP** 5 mins

**SERVES** 4

## INGREDIENTS

2 tbsp reduced-fat mayonnaise
2 tbsp pesto
4 x 15cm (6in) wheat tortillas
100g (3½oz) salad leaves
250g (9oz) sliced turkey breast
6 spring onions, sliced
8 slices cucumber (sliced
    lengthways)
Freshly ground black pepper

1  In a small bowl, combine the mayonnaise and pesto.

2  Spread the pesto mayo evenly on each tortilla.

3  Divide the salad leaves, turkey, spring onions, and cucumber slices between the tortillas, and sprinkle with the black pepper.

4  Roll the tortillas up and cut in half. Enjoy immediately, or wrap and eat them on the go.

**Make ahead:** Prepare the pesto mayo and slice vegetables up to 3 days ahead, and refrigerate for quick assembly.

To lower the fat content, replace the mayonnaise with low fat yogurt. Swap the turkey with chicken strips.

| NUTRITION PER SERVING | | | | |
|---|---|---|---|---|
| ENERGY | 1,008kJ (240kcal) | FAT | 10g |
| CARBOHYDRATES | 22g | CHOLESTEROL | 30mg |
| SUGARS | 3g | SODIUM | 860mg |
| DIETARY FIBRE | 2g | VITAMIN C | 10% |
| PROTEIN | 15g | VITAMIN A | 15% |
| | | IRON | 10% |

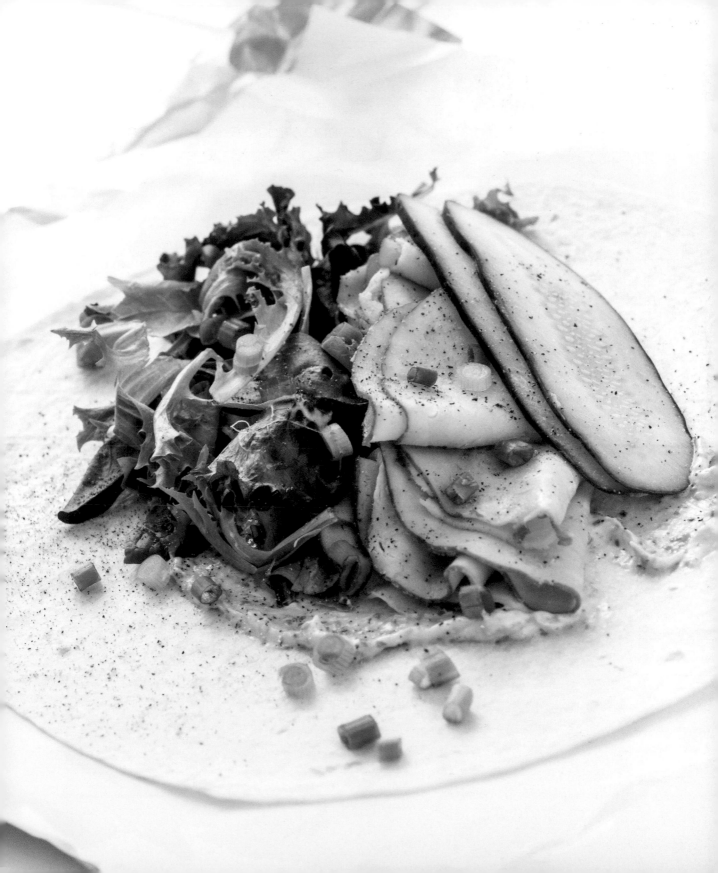

# Egg Drop **Soup**

This classic Asian soup will help hydrate your body and give you a good source of protein at the same time. This is a low carbohydrate option ideal for low workload days or short duration events. Add noodles to increase carbohydrate for higher workload days.

● ○ ○    **Easy**

**PREP** 5 mins
**COOK** 5–10 mins

**SERVES** 2

## INGREDIENTS

1 litre (1¾ pints) low-sodium
   chicken stock
¼ tsp salt
⅛ tsp ground ginger
2 tbsp chopped fresh chives
1½ tbsp cornflour
2 large eggs
1 large egg white

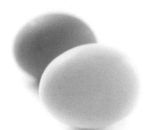

To make this recipe vegetarian, use a low-sodium vegetable stock instead of the chicken stock. Serve with chopped coriander or spring onion.

1  In a large pan over a high heat, heat 780ml (1¼ pints) of the stock. Stir in the salt, ginger, and chives, and bring to the boil.

2  In a small bowl, stir together the remaining chicken stock and cornflour and mix until smooth.

3  In another small bowl, whisk together the eggs and the egg white.

4  Using a fork, drizzle the egg mixture a little at a time into boiling stock mixture.

5  Gradually stir in the cornflour mixture until the soup is the desired consistency.

6  Serve hot.

**Make ahead and freeze:** Prepare up to the end of step 5 up to 6 days ahead. Freeze in individual containers after step 5 for up to 2 months.

| NUTRITION PER SERVING | | | |
|---|---|---|---|
| ENERGY | 462kJ (110kcal) | FAT | 5g |
| CARBOHYDRATES | 3g | CHOLESTEROL | 215mg |
| SUGARS | 0g | SODIUM | 520mg |
| DIETARY FIBRE | 0g | VITAMIN C | 2% |
| PROTEIN | 12g | VITAMIN A | 8% |
| | | IRON | 8% |

# Italian Wedding **Soup**

Enjoy this easy but authentic version of an Italian wedding soup for lunch on busy competition days.

1. In a medium bowl, combine the minced beef, egg, breadcrumbs, Parmesan cheese, basil, and onion powder until well combined. Using your hands, shape the mixture into 2cm (¾in) balls and arrange on a plate.

2. Bring the chicken stock to the boil in a large pan over a medium–high heat. Stir in the endive, orzo pasta, carrots, and the meatballs.

3. Return to the boil, reduce the heat to medium, then simmer, covered, for 10 minutes or until the pasta is al dente. Stir frequently to prevent sticking.

4. Serve hot.

**Make ahead and freeze:** Prepare up to the end of step 3 up to 6 days ahead. Freeze in individual containers after step 3 for up to 2 months.

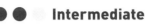 

● ● ○ **Intermediate**

**PREP** 15–20 mins
**COOK** about 15 mins

**SERVES** 4

### INGREDIENTS

225g (8oz) lean minced beef

1 large egg, lightly beaten

2 tbsp dried unseasoned breadcrumbs

1 tbsp grated Parmesan cheese

½ tsp dried basil

½ tsp onion powder

1.3 litres (2¼ pints) low-sodium chicken stock

100g (3½oz) endive, thinly sliced

100g (3½oz) orzo pasta

1 medium carrot, finely chopped

| NUTRITION PER SERVING | | | | |
|---|---|---|---|---|
| ENERGY | 1,092kJ (260kcal) | FAT | 8g |
| CARBOHYDRATES | 26g | CHOLESTEROL | 90mg |
| SUGARS | 2g | SODIUM | 220mg |
| DIETARY FIBRE | 2g | VITAMIN C | 4% |
| PROTEIN | 21g | VITAMIN A | 50% |
| | | IRON | 20% |

# Quick Tortellini **Salad**

You can make this pasta salad well in advance, so you have a handy lunch-to-go on competition day.

● ○ ○   **Easy**

**PREP** 5–10 mins + 2–4 hours marinating
**COOK** 5–10 mins

**SERVES** 6

## INGREDIENTS

500g (1lb 2oz) ready-made three-cheese tortellini

225g (8oz) cherry tomatoes, halved

10g (¼oz) fresh basil, chopped

1 small red onion, chopped

120ml (4fl oz) balsamic vinaigrette dressing

80ml (2½fl oz) water

1 tbsp brown sugar

1 large clove garlic, finely chopped

1   Cook the tortellini according to the packet instructions. Drain and rinse with cold water.

2   In a large bowl, combine the tortellini, cherry tomatoes, basil, and red onion.

3   In a small bowl, combine the balsamic vinaigrette dressing with the water, brown sugar, and garlic. Stir this marinade well until combined.

4   Pour the marinade over the pasta, and toss gently to coat.

5   Cover and refrigerate for at least 2–4 hours.

6   Serve chilled.

**Make ahead:** Refrigerate for 3–5 days.

For an alternative, you could choose tortellini with different fillings. Also, this salad is tasty served warm. Try serving it immediately after preparation or heating it in a microwave-safe container.

| NUTRITION PER SERVING | | | |
|---|---|---|---|
| ENERGY | 1,302kJ (310kcal) | FAT | 9g |
| CARBOHYDRATES | 47g | CHOLESTEROL | 30mg |
| SUGARS | 8g | SODIUM | 540mg |
| DIETARY FIBRE | 3g | VITAMIN C | 10% |
| PROTEIN | 13g | VITAMIN A | 8% |
| | | IRON | 10% |

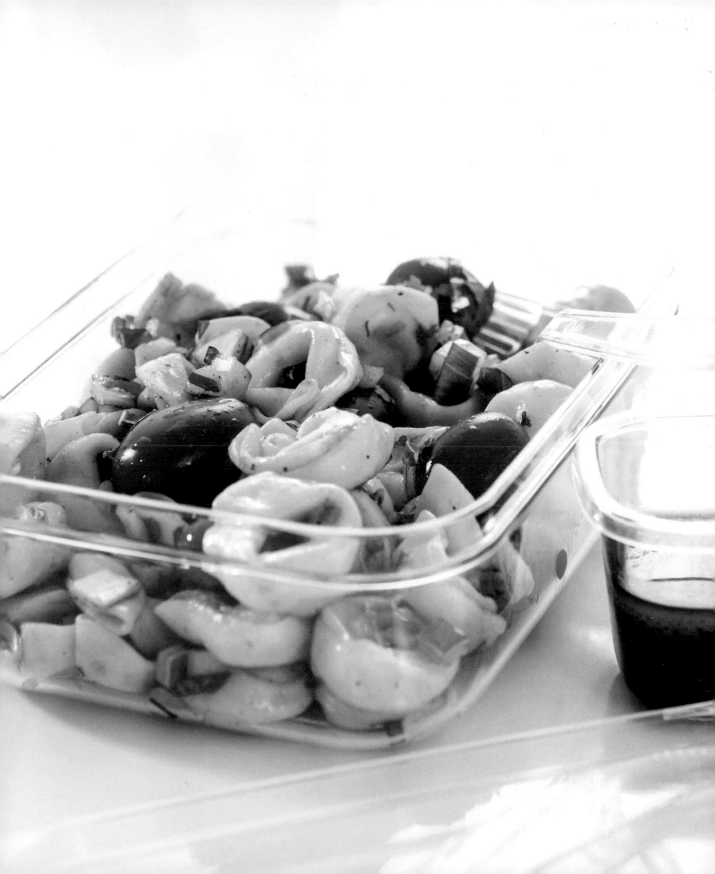

# Greek Pasta **Salad**

This vegetarian dish is packed with vitamin C from the tomatoes, which will enhance the absorption of iron from the spinach.

● ○ ○   **Easy**

**PREP** 10 mins + 1–2 hours
marinating
**COOK** 5–10 mins

**SERVES** 4

**INGREDIENTS**

225g (8oz) tri-colored fusilli pasta

60g (2oz) baby spinach leaves

100g (3½oz) reduced-fat feta
cheese, crumbled

150g (5½oz) cherry tomatoes,
halved

115g (4oz) canned chickpeas,
drained and rinsed

30g (1oz) canned sliced black
olives, drained

4 tsp olive oil

2 tsp lemon juice

2 tsp red wine vinegar

1 tbsp dried oregano

1   In a large pan over a medium–high heat, cook the pasta according to the packet instructions. Drain the cooked pasta, pour into a large bowl, and allow to cool for 5–10 minutes.

2   Mix in the spinach leaves, feta, cherry tomatoes, chickpeas, and black olives.

3   Combine the olive oil, lemon juice, red wine vinegar, and oregano together and stir into the salad lightly until all of the ingredients are coated.

4   Cover the salad and chill for 1–2 hours or until cooled.

5   Enjoy chilled.

**Make ahead:** Refrigerate for 3–5 days.

If you like more dressing, but do not want to increase the oil (and therefore the fat content), add 2 tsp balsamic vinegar and 1 tsp Dijon mustard.

| NUTRITION PER SERVING | | | |
|---|---|---|---|
| ENERGY | 1,516l1kJ (361kcal) | FAT | 10g |
| CARBOHYDRATES | 46g | CHOLESTEROL | 16.5mg |
| SUGARS | 2g | SODIUM | 468mg |
| DIETARY FIBRE | 6g | VITAMIN C | 23% |
| PROTEIN | 15g | VITAMIN A | 24% |
| | | IRON | 19% |

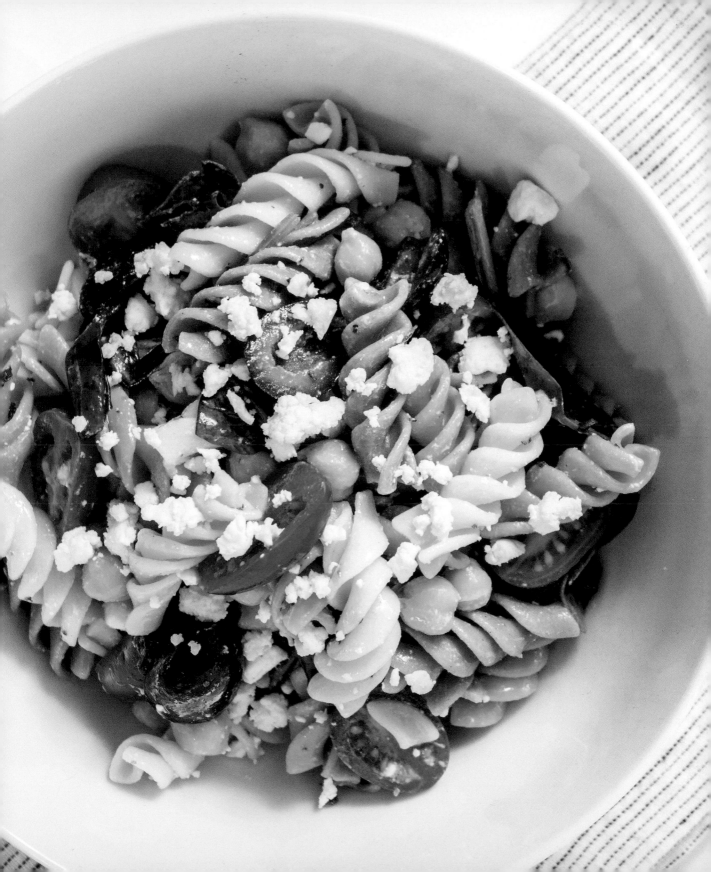

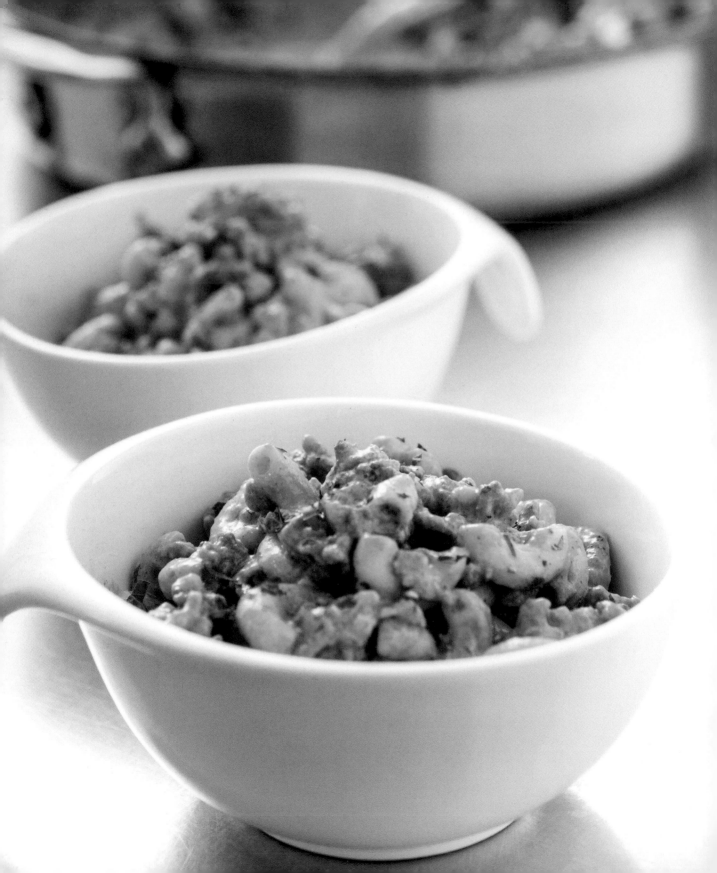

# Spicy Beef and Pasta **Casserole**

An excellent source of protein, this family classic is easy to make. It also contains plenty of carbohydrate to maintain your energy.

1 In a large frying pan over a medium–high heat, cook the minced beef, stirring occasionally, for 5–10 minutes or until the beef is browned. Drain any fat through a colander, and return the beef to the pan.

2 Add the milk, beef stock, elbow macaroni, cornflour, chilli powder, garlic powder, sugar, salt, paprika, and cayenne, and give it a good stir.

3 Bring to the boil, reduce the heat to medium–low, cover, and simmer for 10–12 minutes or until the pasta is al dente.

4 Add the Cheddar cheese, and stir until combined.

5 Garnish with parsley, and serve hot.

**Make ahead and freeze:** Freeze after step 4 for up to 2 months. Thaw in the refrigerator for 1 or 2 days before baking at 180°C (350°F/gas 4) for about 45 minutes or until cooked through.

**Storage:** Refrigerate leftovers for 3–5 days.

● ○ ○ ○　**Easy**

**PREP** 5–10 mins
**COOK** about 22 mins

**SERVES** 6

## INGREDIENTS

450g (1lb) lean minced beef

600ml (1 pint) whole milk

240ml (8fl oz) low-sodium beef stock

210g (7½oz) elbow macaroni

1 tbsp cornflour

1 tbsp chilli powder

2 tsp garlic powder

1 tsp granulated sugar

1 tsp salt

¾ tsp paprika

¼ tsp cayenne pepper

225g (8oz) Cheddar cheese, grated

Fresh parsley, to garnish

| NUTRITION PER SERVING | | | |
|---|---|---|---|
| ENERGY | 1,680kJ (400kcal) | FAT | 13g |
| CARBOHYDRATES | 34g | CHOLESTEROL | 65mg |
| SUGARS | 6g | SODIUM | 420mg |
| DIETARY FIBRE | 35g | VITAMIN C | 2% |
| PROTEIN | 35g | VITAMIN A | 5% |
| | | IRON | 20% |

To lower the fat more, use the same amount of minced chicken or lean minced turkey instead of the minced beef. You can also use reduced-fat Cheddar and semi-skimmed milk.

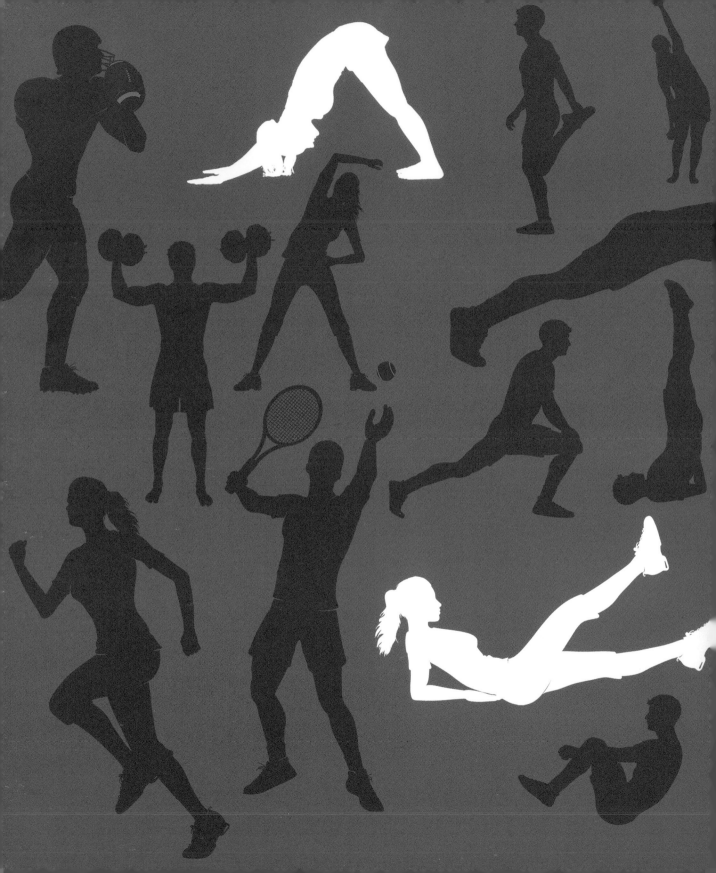

# Recipes for
# **Recovery**

Now that your competition or training session is over, it's time to let your body recover. To help with that, in Part 4, we share some tasty and easy-to-prepare recovery recipes, including high-carbohydrate, protein containing recovery drinks and carry-along portable foods for eating immediately afterwards, as well as soups, salads, mains, side dishes, and desserts meant to help your body restock its nutrients and get you ready for the next big event.

To save time, in this section we offer good, homemade alternatives to shop-bought foods that are quick and easy to prepare.

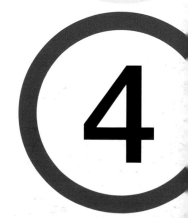

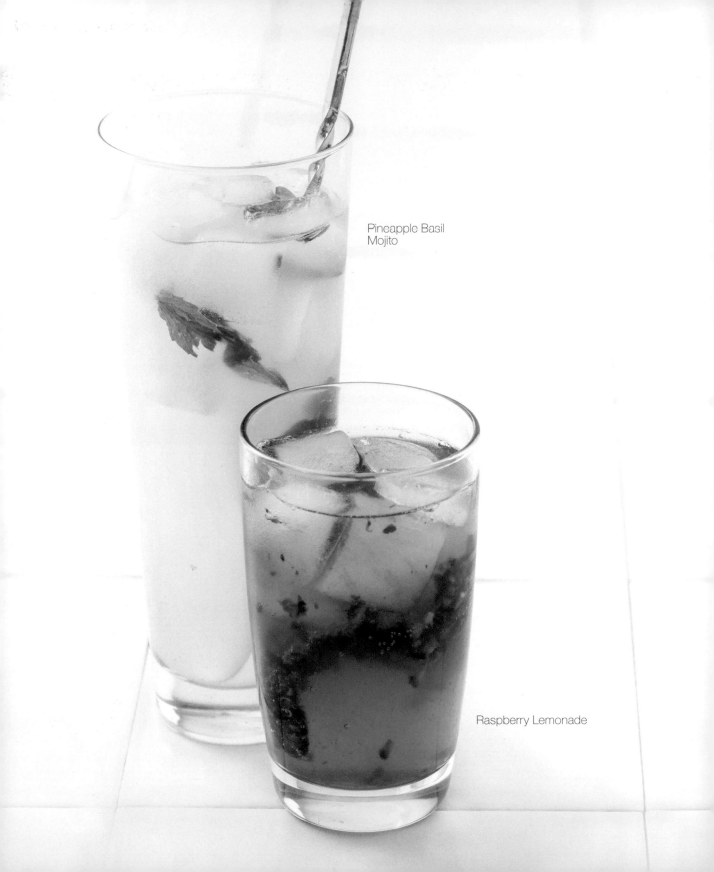

Pineapple Basil
Mojito

Raspberry Lemonade

# Pineapple Basil **Mojito**

This sweet and delicious summery recovery "mocktail" is perfect for providing fluid and carbohydrate for recovery after a workout or competition.

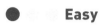 **Easy**

**PREP** 5 mins

**SERVES** 1

## INGREDIENTS

1 tbsp granulated sugar
⅛ tsp salt
3 fresh basil leaves
120ml (4fl oz) pineapple juice
120ml (4fl oz) limeade
180ml (6fl oz) water

1  In a large glass, combine the sugar, salt, and basil leaves. Press the ingredients together with the back of a spoon, until the basil leaves look a little bruised.

2  Add the pineapple juice, limeade, and water, and stir to combine.

3  Drink immediately over ice.

| NUTRITION PER SERVING | | | |
|---|---|---|---|
| **ENERGY** 714kJ (170kcal) | | **FAT** | 0g |
| **CARBOHYDRATES** | 42g | **CHOLESTEROL** | 0mg |
| **SUGARS** | 41g | **SODIUM** | 300mg |
| **DIETARY FIBRE** | 0g | **VITAMIN C** | 20% |
| **PROTEIN** | 0g | **VITAMIN A** | 0% |
| | | **IRON** | 2% |

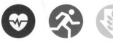

# Raspberry **Lemonade**

This beautifully pink drink combines sweet raspberries with tart lemon juice to make a fabulously refreshing drink. It's a good source of vitamin C.

● **Easy**

**PREP** 2 mins

**SERVES** 1

## INGREDIENTS

5 fresh raspberries
120ml (4fl oz) water
Juice of ½ lemon (about 1 tbsp)
1 tbsp runny honey
4 tbsp coconut water

1  Place the fresh raspberries in a bottle, and crush slightly with the back of a spoon.

2  Add the water, lemon juice, honey, and coconut water, and shake vigorously for about 30 seconds or until combined.

3  Serve over ice.

| NUTRITION PER SERVING | | | |
|---|---|---|---|
| **ENERGY** 420kJ (100kcal) | | **FAT** | 0g |
| **CARBOHYDRATES** | 26g | **CHOLESTEROL** | 0mg |
| **SUGARS** | 18g | **SODIUM** | 65mg |
| **DIETARY FIBRE** | 1g | **VITAMIN C** | 35% |
| **PROTEIN** | 1g | **VITAMIN A** | 0% |
| | | **IRON** | 2% |

# Blueberry Lavender
# **Lemonade**

This is a light and refreshing lemonade that provides fluid and carbohydrate for recovery.

● ● ○   **Intermediate**

**PREP** 15 mins
**COOK** 5 mins

## SERVES 1

## INGREDIENTS

2 tbsp granulated sugar

2 tbsp water

2 tbsp dried lavender flowers

1/8 tsp salt

30g (1oz) fresh blueberries

Juice of 2 medium lemons

240ml (8fl oz) cold water

**1**    In a pan over a medium heat, simmer the sugar and water for about 5 minutes.

**2**    Place the dried lavender flowers in a medium bowl, add the sugar water, and set aside for 1–2 hours. Strain the lavender-flavoured water through a sieve.

**3**    In a large glass, crush the salt with the blueberries slightly. Add the lavender water, lemon juice, and cold water, and stir to mix well.

**4**    Serve over ice or chilled.

| NUTRITION PER SERVING | | | |
|---|---|---|---|
| **ENERGY** 564kJ (130kcal) | | FAT | 0g |
| **CARBOHYDRATES** | 34g | CHOLESTEROL | 0mg |
| **SUGARS** | 28g | SODIUM | 300mg |
| **DIETARY FIBRE** | 2g | VITAMIN C | 60% |
| **PROTEIN** | 0g | VITAMIN A | 2% |
| | | IRON | 2% |

# Gingerade

This light thirst-quencher contains soothing ginger – perfect to cool you off after a strenuous workout.

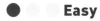 **Easy**

---

**PREP** 5 mins

---

**SERVES** 1

---

**INGREDIENTS**

175ml (6fl oz) ginger ale
120ml (4fl oz) prepared lemonade
120ml (4fl oz) sparkling water
⅛ tsp salt

1 Combine all the ingredients together in a water bottle and shake well.

2 Drink over ice.

| NUTRITION PER SERVING | | | |
|---|---|---|---|
| **ENERGY** | 504kJ (120kcal) | **FAT** | 0g |
| **CARBOHYDRATES** | 30g | **CHOLESTEROL** | 0mg |
| **SUGARS** | 29g | **SODIUM** | 310mg |
| **DIETARY FIBRE** | 0g | **VITAMIN C** | 0% |
| **PROTEIN** | 0g | **VITAMIN A** | 0% |
| | | **IRON** | 0% |

# Blueberry Banana
# **Recovery Smoothie**

This simple, light, and creamy vegan smoothie is perfect for when you don't have an appetite.

● ◌ ◌ **Easy**

**PREP** 1 min

**SERVES** 2

## INGREDIENTS

1 small banana, peeled and sliced

150g (5½oz) fresh blueberries

240ml (8fl oz) almond milk

1 tbsp granulated sugar

120ml (4fl oz) ice cubes

**1**  Combine all the ingredients in a blender for about 1 minute, or until completely combined.

**2**  Drink immediately.

> To increase protein and lower fat, use semi-skimmed cow milk or soy milk instead of almond milk.

| NUTRITION PER SERVING | | | |
|---|---|---|---|
| ENERGY  420kJ (100kcal) | | FAT | 1.5g |
| CARBOHYDRATES | 23g | CHOLESTEROL | 0mg |
| SUGARS | 17g | SODIUM | 50mg |
| DIETARY FIBRE | 2g | VITAMIN C | 110% |
| PROTEIN | 1g | VITAMIN A | 4% |
| | | IRON | 2% |

# Kiwi Pineapple
# **Chia Smoothie**

Reach for this excellent recovery smoothie after an intense workout or a match. Chia seeds are rich in fibre, and are a source of calcium and omega 3 fatty acids.

● ◌ ◌ **Easy**

**PREP** 5 mins

**SERVES** 3

## INGREDIENTS

60g (2oz) fresh spinach

3 large kiwis, peeled and sliced

1 small banana, peeled and sliced

120ml (4fl oz) low fat plain yogurt

4 tbsp fresh pineapple, chopped

4 tbsp fresh orange juice

1 tbsp chia seeds

**1**  Combine all the ingredients in a blender for about 1 minute, or until completely combined.

**2**  Drink immediately.

| NUTRITION PER SERVING | | | |
|---|---|---|---|
| ENERGY  622kJ (148kcal) | | FAT | 2.9g |
| CARBOHYDRATES | 23g | CHOLESTEROL | 3.3mg |
| SUGARS | 17g | SODIUM | 46mg |
| DIETARY FIBRE | 4.9g | VITAMIN C | 118% |
| PROTEIN | 4.2g | VITAMIN A | 19% |
| | | IRON | 11% |

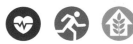

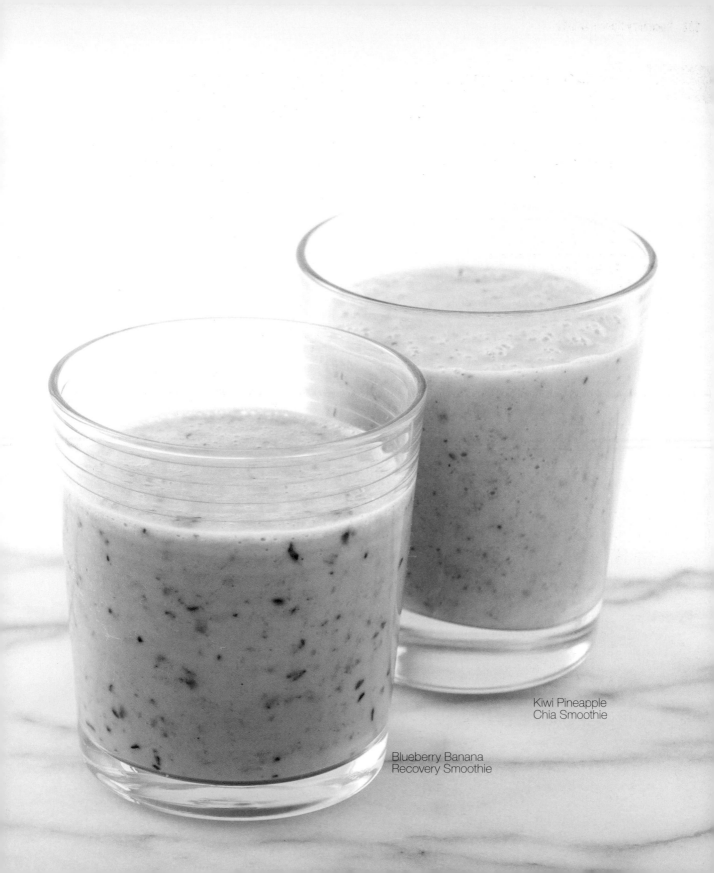

Kiwi Pineapple
Chia Smoothie

Blueberry Banana
Recovery Smoothie

# Peaches and Cream
# **Smoothie**

This thick and creamy smoothie is a source of protein, providing 16 grams per serving to help muscles recover.

● ○ ○ **Easy**

**PREP** 5–10 mins

**SERVES** 1

## INGREDIENTS

120ml (4fl oz) whole milk
60ml (2fl oz) vanilla Greek yogurt
60g (2oz) low-fat cottage cheese
2 tsp sugar
Juice of 2 medium oranges
190g (6½oz) frozen peaches

**1**  Combine all the ingredients together in a blender for 1 minute or until smooth.

**2**  Drink immediately.

> If you do not tolerate dairy or you are vegan, use soy milk instead of milk and 60g silken tofu instead of yogurt.

| NUTRITION PER SERVING | | | |
|---|---|---|---|
| **ENERGY** 1,176kJ (280kcal) | | **FAT** | 9g |
| **CARBOHYDRATES** | 35g | **CHOLESTEROL** | 20mg |
| **SUGARS** | 34g | **SODIUM** | 300mg |
| **DIETARY FIBRE** | 2g | **VITAMIN C** | 160% |
| **PROTEIN** | 16g | **VITAMIN A** | 10% |
| | | **IRON** | 2% |

# Green Monster
# **Smoothie**

This superb green smoothie contains protein and carbohydrate and the spinach is high in antioxidants. Perfect to have before or between competitions.

● ○ ○ **Easy**

**PREP** 5 mins

**SERVES** 1

## INGREDIENTS

120ml (4fl oz) semi-skimmed milk
120ml (4fl oz) low fat plain yogurt
1 small banana, peeled, frozen, and sliced
2 tsp creamy peanut or nut butter
60g (2oz) fresh spinach
240ml (8fl oz) ice cubes

**1**  Combine all the ingredients together in a blender for 1 minute or until smooth.

**2**  Drink immediately.

| NUTRITION PER SERVING | | | |
|---|---|---|---|
| **ENERGY** 1,088kJ (259kcal) | | **FAT** | 10g |
| **CARBOHYDRATES** | 25g | **CHOLESTEROL** | 18mg |
| **SUGARS** | 20g | **SODIUM** | 230mg |
| **DIETARY FIBRE** | 3g | **VITAMIN C** | 31% |
| **PROTEIN** | 14g | **VITAMIN A** | 58% |
| | | **IRON** | 16% |

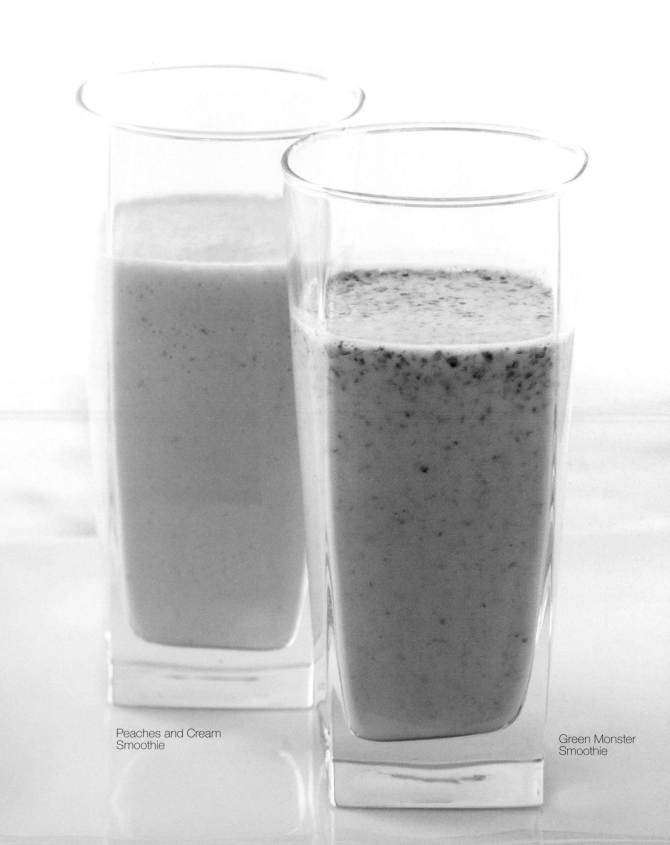

Peaches and Cream
Smoothie

Green Monster
Smoothie

# Reduced-Fat **Tuna Melts**

Crave the classic tuna melt but don't want all the fat? This much lighter version is full of protein and carbohydrate, and lower in fat.

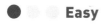

● ○ ○   **Easy**

**PREP** 10 mins
**COOK** 3–5 mins

**SERVES** 4

## INGREDIENTS

2 x 160g (5¾oz) tins tuna chunks in water, drained

½ small red onion, diced

2 tbsp reduced-fat mayonnaise

Juice of ½ medium lemon (about 1 tbsp)

1 tbsp fresh parsley, chopped

⅛ tsp salt

1 tsp Dijon or wholegrain mustard

⅛ tsp freshly ground black pepper

4 slices wholemeal bread, toasted

2 large tomatoes, sliced

100g (3½oz) sharp Cheddar cheese, grated

To further lower the fat content of the melt, replace the cheese with mozzarella or reduced fat cheese.

1  Preheat the grill.

2  Meanwhile, in a medium bowl, combine the tuna, red onion, mayonnaise, lemon juice, parsley, salt, mustard, and black pepper.

3  Spread one-quarter of the tuna mixture on each slice of toasted wholemeal bread, and top with slices of tomatoes and sharp Cheddar cheese.

4  Place the sandwiches on a baking sheet, and grill for 3–5 minutes or until the cheese is bubbling and starting to turn golden brown.

5  Serve immediately, or allow to cool and wrap in greaseproof paper and kitchen foil for later.

**Make ahead:** Refrigerate after step 2 for up to 3 days for quicker assembly.

| NUTRITION PER SERVING | | | |
|---|---|---|---|
| ENERGY | 1302kJ (310kcal) | FAT | 13g |
| CARBOHYDRATES | 26g | CHOLESTEROL | 70mg |
| SUGARS | 5g | SODIUM | 800mg |
| DIETARY FIBRE | 8g | VITAMIN C | 15% |
| PROTEIN | 29g | VITAMIN A | 15% |
| | | IRON | 6% |

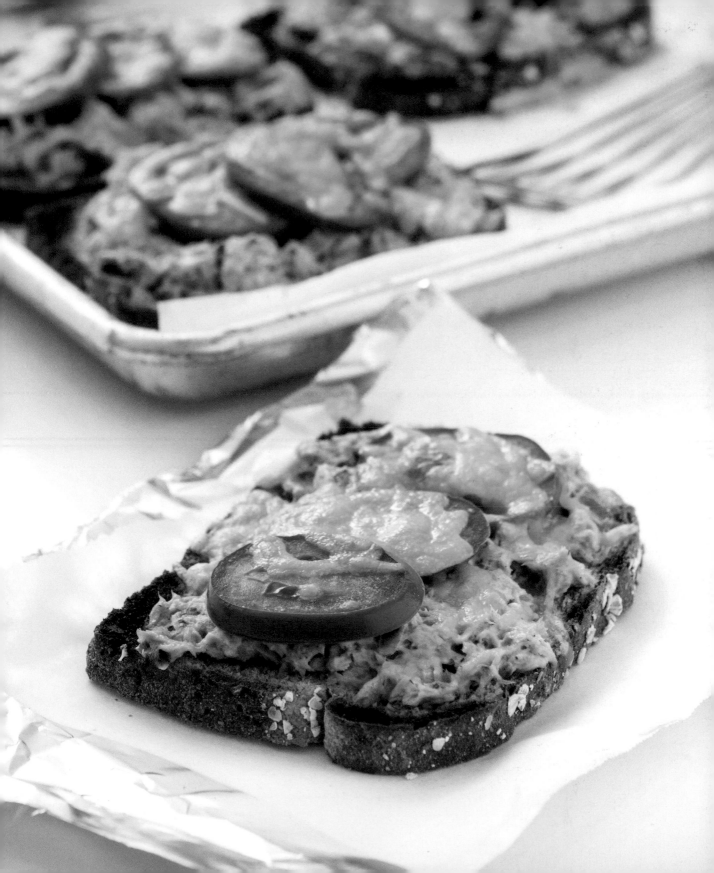

# Mediterranean Salmon **Wraps**

Wrap up grilled salmon and a couscous salad, flavoured with delicious fresh herbs, vegetables, and citrus, in a tortilla – it makes a nutritious and flavoursome meal on-the-go.

● ● ● **Easy**

**PREP** 10 mins
**COOK** 16–20 mins

**SERVES** 4

## INGREDIENTS

4 x 115g (4oz) skinless salmon
  fillets
80ml (2¾fl oz) water
55g (scant 2oz) couscous
15g (½oz) sun-dried tomatoes
60g (2oz) fresh parsley, chopped
12g (½oz) fresh mint, chopped
Juice of 2 medium lemons
1 tbsp extra-virgin olive oil
2 tsp garlic, finely chopped
¼ tsp salt
¼ tsp freshly ground
  black pepper
4 x 25cm (10in) wheat tortillas
4 leaves red leaf lettuce
1 medium cucumber, sliced into
  chunky matchsticks

1  Set a medium frying pan over a medium heat, and lightly spray it with cooking spray.

2  Place the salmon fillets in the pan, and cook for 6–8 minutes on each side or until the fish flakes easily. Remove from the pan, and set aside.

3  Meanwhile, bring water to the boil in a small saucepan over a medium–high heat. Tip in the couscous, stir, and remove the pan from heat.

4  Add the sun-dried tomatoes, cover, and allow to sit for 5 minutes. Fluff with a fork, and set aside.

5  In a small bowl, combine the parsley, mint, lemon juice, extra-virgin olive oil, garlic, salt, and black pepper. Add to the couscous, stir through, and set aside.

6  Evenly divide the couscous mixture between the tortillas, spread into a thin layer, and top with the red leaf lettuce. Divide the salmon between the wraps, and top with cucumber slices. Roll up each wrap, just like a burrito, cut in half, and enjoy warm or chilled.

**Make ahead:** Prepare up to 3 days ahead, and refrigerate.

| NUTRITION PER SERVING | | | |
|---|---|---|---|
| ENERGY | 2,447kJ (583kcal) | FAT | 23.5g |
| CARBOHYDRATES | 60g | CHOLESTEROL | 60mg |
| SUGARS | 2g | SODIUM | 640mg |
| DIETARY FIBRE | 4g | VITAMIN C | 60% |
| PROTEIN | 33g | VITAMIN A | 30% |
| | | IRON | 25% |

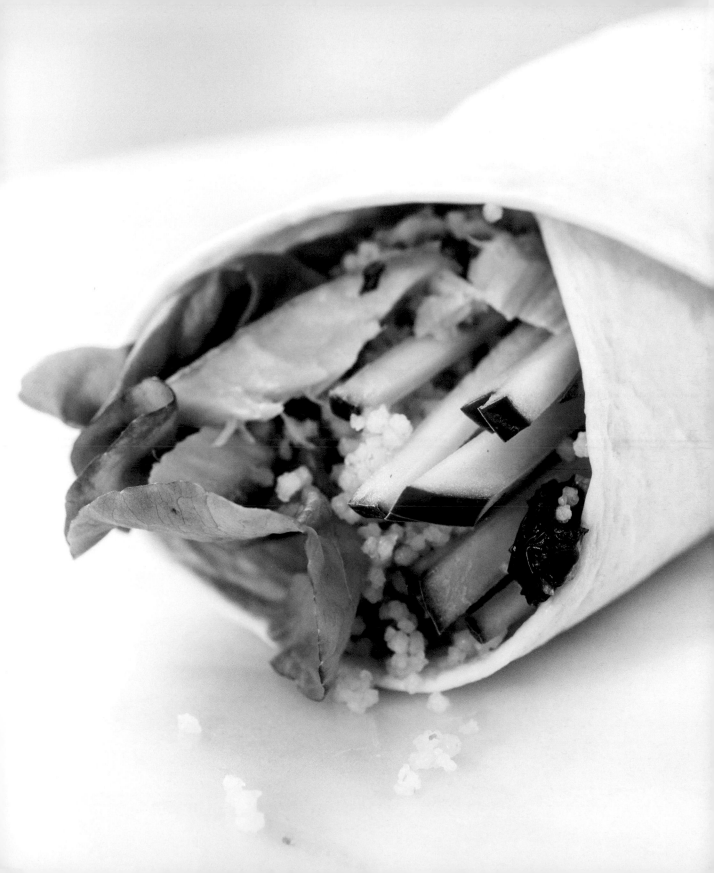

# Easy Slow Cooker Pumpkin Pie
# **Rice Pudding**

This warm and filling treat is easy to prepare in the colder months to get in a few extra carbs. That said, it is tasty eaten warm or cold.

● ◌ ◌ ◌  **Easy**

**PREP** 5 mins
**COOK** about 5 hours

**SERVES** 10

## INGREDIENTS

185g (6½oz) short-grain white rice (not quick cooking)

350ml (12fl oz) light evaporated milk

490g (1lb 1oz) tinned pumpkin

780ml (1⅓ pints) whole milk

85g (3oz) light brown sugar

1 tbsp pumpkin pie spice

¼ tsp salt

1 tsp vanilla extract

60g (2oz) raisins

1  Lightly coat the inside of a 3-litre (5¼ pints) slow cooker with cooking spray.

2  In the slow cooker, combine the rice, evaporated milk, pumpkin, milk, brown sugar, pumpkin pie spice, salt, vanilla extract, and raisins.

3  Cover, and cook on low for about 5 hours or until the rice is tender.

4  Serve warm rather than hot.

**Storage:** Refrigerate leftovers for 3–5 days.

| NUTRITION PER SERVING | | | |
|---|---|---|---|
| ENERGY | 1,218kJ (290kcal) | FAT | 2g |
| CARBOHYDRATES | 60g | CHOLESTEROL | 5mg |
| SUGARS | 26g | SODIUM | 135mg |
| DIETARY FIBRE | 4g | VITAMIN C | 0% |
| PROTEIN | 8g | VITAMIN A | 140% |
| | | IRON | 15% |

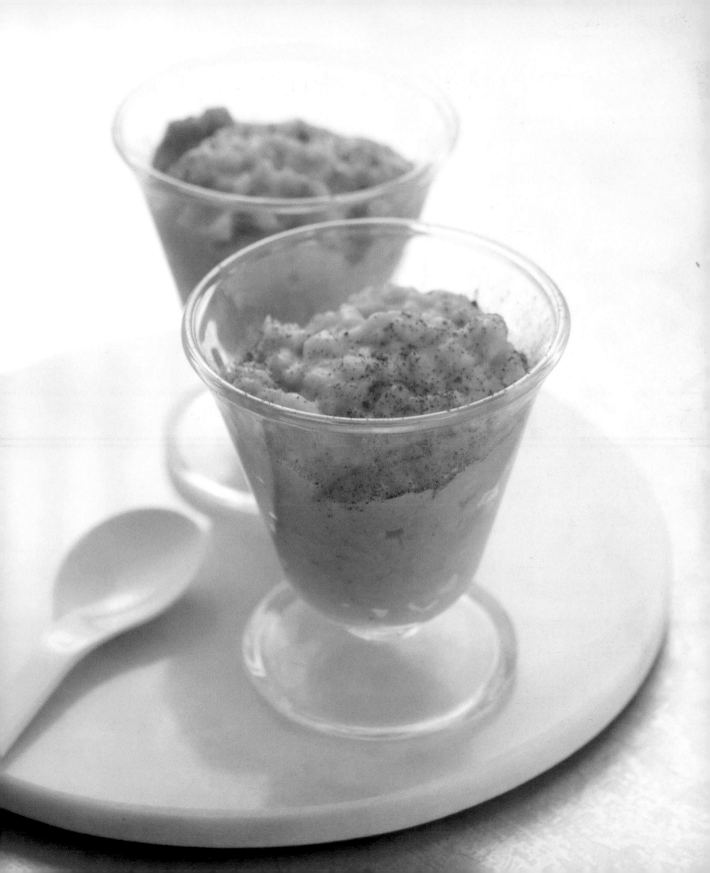

# Vegetable **Stew**

A quick an easy vegetarian vegetable stew that is ideal for warming you up on a cold winter's day and when you need to get in extra carbs and vegetables to refuel.

● ○ ○   **Easy**

**PREP** 10 mins
**COOK** about 30 mins

**SERVES** 4

## INGREDIENTS

1 tbsp extra-virgin olive oil

1 medium sweet onion, diced

2 medium carrots, peeled
  and diced

2 medium parsnips, peeled
  and diced

2 medium celery stalks, diced

720ml (1¼ pints) vegetable stock

480g (1lb 1oz) tinned chopped
  tomatoes, drained

85g (3oz) tomato purée

480g (1lb 1oz) tinned butter
  beans, drained and rinsed

30g (1oz) fresh parsley, chopped

1   Heat the oil in a medium pan over a medium heat. Add the onion and cook for about 5 minutes or until translucent.

2   Add the carrots, parsnips, and celery to the pan, cover, and cook for about 5 minutes.

3   Add the vegetable stock, tomatoes, and tomato purée to the pan, and bring to the boil.

4   Cover, reduce heat to medium–low, and simmer for about 10 minutes.

5   Stir in the butter beans, and cook for a further 5 minutes or until the vegetables are tender.

6   Stir in the parsley, and serve hot.

**Make ahead and freeze:** Prepare up to the end of step 5 up to 6 days ahead. Freeze in individual containers after step 5 for up to 2 months.

To bulk up the protein content of this recipe, brown 350g (12oz) skinless chicken with the onion.

| NUTRITION PER SERVING | | | |
|---|---|---|---|
| ENERGY | 1,008kJ (240kcal) | FAT | 4g |
| CARBOHYDRATES | 48g | CHOLESTEROL | 0mg |
| SUGARS | 17g | SODIUM | 1,280mg |
| DIETARY FIBRE | 12g | VITAMIN C | 70% |
| PROTEIN | 10g | VITAMIN A | 160% |
| | | IRON | 25% |

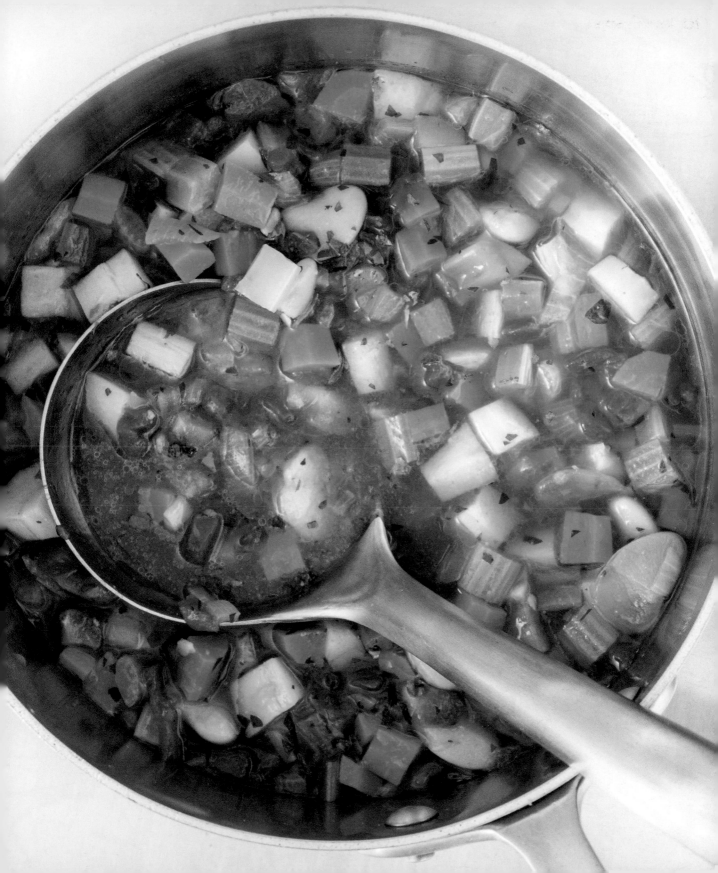

# Hearty Legume and Beef **Soup**

This filling soup is just bursting with flavour. It's excellent for warming you up after time spent competing outside in the cold.

 **Easy**

**PREP** 10–15 mins
**COOK** about 45 mins

**SERVES** 2

## INGREDIENTS

250g (9oz) lean beef or lamb
1 tsp oil
1 medium carrot, diced
1 medium celery stalk, diced
1 small white onion, chopped
480ml (15½fl oz) low-sodium
    beef stock
350ml (12fl oz) amber beer
1 tbsp fresh basil leaves
¼ tsp freshly ground
    black pepper
1 bay leaf
2 tbsp grated Parmesan cheese

1   In a large pan over a medium–high heat, brown the meat, carrot, celery and onion in oil.

2   In a separate pot, bring the beef stock, beer, and lentils to the boil. Reduce the heat to medium–low, cover, and simmer, stirring occasionally, for 20–25 minutes or until the lentils are tender.

3   Stir in the lean beef, carrot, celery, onion, basil, black pepper, and bay leaf. Cover, and simmer, stirring occasionally, for 20 minutes. Remove the bay leaf.

4   Serve hot with Parmesan cheese sprinkled on top.

**Make ahead and freeze:** Prepare up to the end of step 2 up to 6 days ahead. Freeze in individual containers after step 2 for up to 2 months.

| NUTRITION PER SERVING | | | |
|---|---|---|---|
| ENERGY | 2,352kJ (560kcal) | FAT | 21g |
| CARBOHYDRATES | 31g | CHOLESTEROL | 95mg |
| SUGARS | 4.6g | SODIUM | 690mg |
| DIETARY FIBRE | 9.5g | VITAMIN C | 10% |
| PROTEIN | 38g | VITAMIN A | 130% |
| | | IRON | 25% |

# Turkey **Chilli**

Move over beef – try this wonderful spicy turkey chilli. It is a good source of protein and rich in flavour.

**1** Heat the oil in a large pan over a medium heat. Add the red pepper, onion, and garlic, and cook, stirring occasionally, for 5–8 minutes or until the vegetables have softened.

**2** Increase the heat to medium–high, add the turkey, and cook, breaking up the meat into smaller pieces with a spoon, for 4–6 minutes or until the turkey is no longer pink and is cooked through.

**3** Add the chilli powder, salt, oregano, cumin, cayenne, and cinnamon, and cook, stirring occasionally, for 1 minute.

**4** Add the tomatoes with their juice and the vegetable stock, and bring to a simmer.

**5** Add the cannellini beans, return to a simmer, reduce the heat to medium–low, and add the bay leaf. Simmer, stirring occasionally, for about 30 minutes.

**6** Remove the bay leaf and serve hot.

**Make ahead and freeze:** Prepare up to the end of step 5 up to 6 days ahead. Freeze in individual containers after step 5 for up to 2 months.

● **Easy**

**PREP** 10 mins
**COOK** 45 mins

**SERVES** 6

**INGREDIENTS**

2 tbsp extra-virgin olive oil

1 medium red pepper, deseeded and diced

1 yellow onion, diced

2 cloves garlic, finely chopped

450g (1lb) lean turkey mince

3 tbsp chilli powder

2 tsp salt

½ tsp dried oregano

½ tsp ground cumin

⅛ tsp cayenne pepper

⅛ tsp ground cinnamon

800g (28oz) tinned chopped tomatoes, with juice

240ml (8fl oz) low-sodium vegetable stock

800g (28oz) tinned cannellini beans, drained and rinsed

1 bay leaf

To lower the sodium, omit the salt, use dried beans (the preparation will change), or pick low-sodium beans and tomatoes, drained and rinsed.

| NUTRITION PER SERVING | | | |
|---|---|---|---|
| ENERGY | 1,302kJ (310kcal) | FAT | 10g |
| CARBOHYDRATES | 32g | CHOLESTEROL | 45mg |
| SUGARS | 8g | SODIUM | 1,530mg |
| DIETARY FIBRE | 9g | VITAMIN C | 70% |
| PROTEIN | 25g | VITAMIN A | 40% |
| | | IRON | 25% |

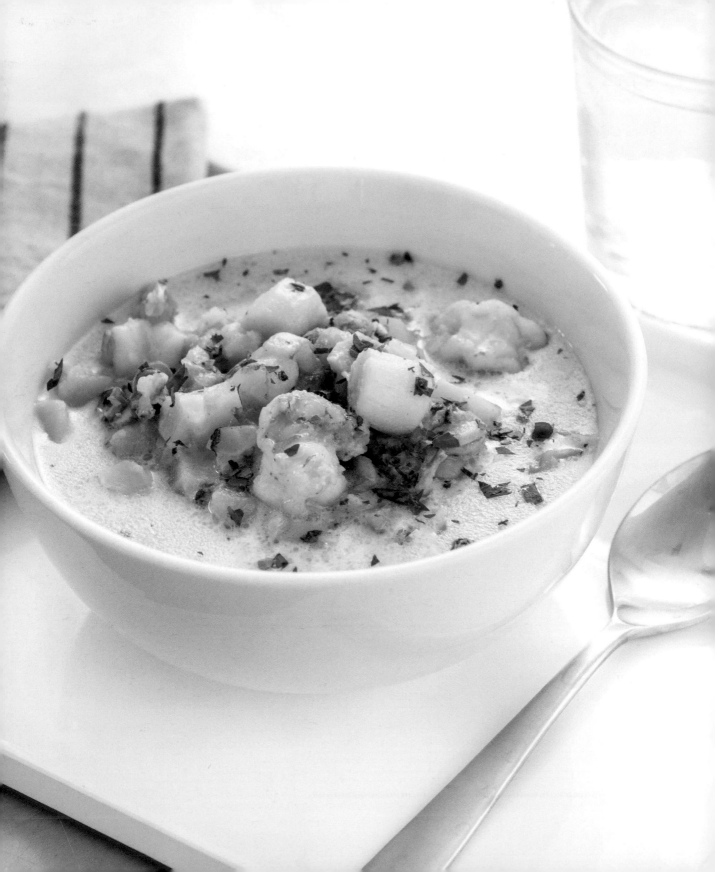

# Seafood **Chowder**

This chowder is a hearty meal that you can enjoy with your whole family. Like all seafood, oysters are a good source of zinc and iron.

**1** In a large pan over a medium heat, cook the bacon for 2–5 minutes or until browned.

**2** Add the onions and cook for 10 minutes.

**3** Sprinkle in the flour and stir until well combined.

**4** Next, add the clam juice, potatoes, thyme, salt, and black pepper. Bring to a simmer, and cook for about 10 minutes or until the potatoes are almost fork-tender.

**5** Add the clams, haddock, prawns, scallops, and oysters, and simmer for 10 minutes.

**6** Pour in the milk and heat through.

**7** Serve immediately.

**Make ahead and freeze:** Prepare up to the end of step 6 up to 6 days ahead. Freeze in individual containers after step 6 for up to 2 months.

● ● ●   **Easy**

**PREP** 20 mins
**COOK** 45 mins

**SERVES** 12

**INGREDIENTS**

175g (6oz) streaky bacon, cut into 1cm (½in) pieces

2 large yellow onions, diced

60g (2oz) plain flour

480ml (16fl oz) clam juice

4 medium white potatoes, peeled and diced

1½ tsp fresh thyme

1 tsp salt

½ tsp freshly cracked black pepper

225g (8oz) shucked clams

225g (8oz) haddock, cut into 2cm (¾in) chunks

225g (8oz) prawns, peeled and deveined

225g (8oz) scallops

225g (8oz) shucked oysters

1 litre (1¾ pints) whole milk

Lower the fat content by replacing whole milk with semi-skimmed milk and replacing the bacon with lean ham.

| NUTRITION PER SERVING | | | |
|---|---|---|---|
| ENERGY | 1,050kJ (250kcal) | FAT | 9g |
| CARBOHYDRATES | 22g | CHOLESTEROL | 80mg |
| SUGARS | 6g | SODIUM | 570mg |
| DIETARY FIBRE | 2g | VITAMIN C | 20% |
| PROTEIN | 20g | VITAMIN A | 4% |
| | | IRON | 30% |

# Easy Minestrone **Soup**

This meat-free soup is jam packed with a rainbow of vegetables.
It will warm you up and keep you moving.

● ○ ○ ○ **Easy**

**PREP** 15 mins
**COOK** about 40 mins

**SERVES** 4

## INGREDIENTS

2 tbsp extra-virgin olive oil

1 small white onion, chopped

3 cloves garlic, finely chopped

2 medium celery stalks, rinsed
  and diced

1 medium courgette, diced

1 cup fresh green beans, cut into
  1cm (½in) pieces

1 medium carrot, peeled and
  diced

800g (1¾lb) tinned chopped
  tomatoes, with juice

1 litre (1¾ pints) reduced-sodium
  vegetable stock

480ml (16fl oz) water

400g (14oz) tinned cannellini
  beans, rinsed and drained

100g (3½oz) elbow macaroni

½ tsp dried oregano

1 tsp dried basil

¼ tsp salt

½ tsp freshly ground black
  pepper

25g (scant 1oz) Parmesan
  cheese, grated

Small handful spinach leaves,
  sliced finely (optional)

1  Heat the oil in a large pan over a medium heat.

2  Add the onion, garlic, and celery, and cook for 5 minutes,
   or until lightly browned.

3  Add the courgette, green beans, carrot, and chopped
   tomatoes and juice, and cook for a further 1–2 minutes.

4  Stir in the vegetable stock, water, cannellini beans,
   macaroni, oregano, basil, salt, and black pepper, then
   simmer for 25–30 minutes, or until the vegetables and
   macaroni are tender.

5  Stir in the Parmesan cheese and serve hot, garnished
   with the finely sliced spinach leaves, if desired.

**Make ahead and freeze:** Prepare up to the end
of step 4 up to 6 days ahead. Freeze in individual
containers after step 4 for up to 2 months.

| NUTRITION PER SERVING | | | |
|---|---|---|---|
| ENERGY | 1,470kJ (350kcal) | FAT | 5.3g |
| CARBOHYDRATES | 52g | CHOLESTEROL | 5mg |
| SUGARS | 13g | SODIUM | 860mg |
| DIETARY FIBRE | 10g | VITAMIN C | 60% |
| PROTEIN | 14g | VITAMIN A | 90% |
| | | IRON | 20% |

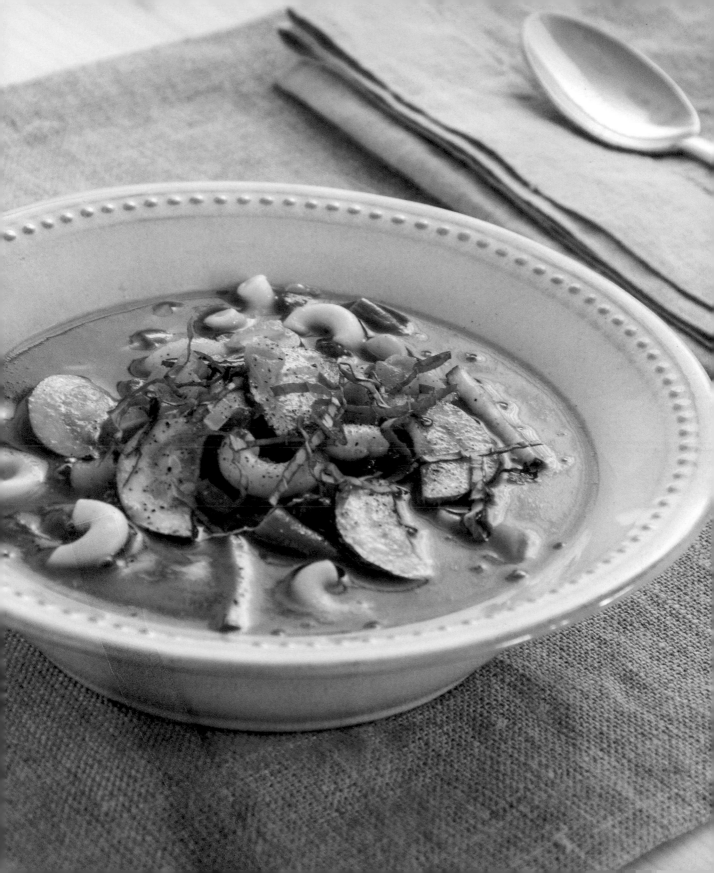

# Mediterranean **Quinoa Salad**

This Greek-style vegetable salad is just right for a quick bite after the gym or a match. Quinoa is a wholegrain, and therefore high in fibre. Serve with chicken for a balanced meal.

● ○ ○ **Easy**

**PREP** 10 mins
**COOK** 15 mins + 1–2hours cooling

**SERVES** 6

## INGREDIENTS

190g (6¾oz) quinoa
480ml (15½fl oz) water
1 small red onion, diced
Juice of 1 medium lemon (2tbsp)
30g (1oz) kalamata olives, pitted and sliced
1 tbsp extra-virgin olive oil
2 medium cucumbers, peeled, deseeded, and diced
150g (5½oz) cherry tomatoes, halved
50g (1¾oz) feta cheese, crumbled
15g (½oz) fresh parsley, chopped
1 tsp salt
½ tsp freshly ground black pepper

1 Rinse the quinoa thoroughly for about 30 seconds.

2 In a medium pan over a medium–high heat, bring the water and the quinoa to the boil. Reduce the heat to low, cover, and simmer for 15 minutes.

3 Remove from the heat, and keep the quinoa covered for 5 minutes.

4 Fluff up the quinoa with a fork, and pour into a large bowl to cool for 10–15 minutes.

5 Add the onion, lemon juice, olives, extra-virgin olive oil, cucumber, cherry tomatoes, feta, parsley, salt, and black pepper, and stir to combine.

6 Refrigerate for 1–2 hours before serving.

**Make ahead:** Prepare up to 3–5 days ahead, and refrigerate.

For a lower fat version, replace with reduced fat feta cheese. For an Italian twist, swap the feta for 60g (2oz) diced fresh mozzarella and add chopped fresh basil.

| NUTRITION PER SERVING | | | |
|---|---|---|---|
| ENERGY | 746kJ (178kcal) | FAT | 6.5g |
| CARBOHYDRATES | 24g | CHOLESTEROL | 0mg |
| SUGARS | 4g | SODIUM | 650mg |
| DIETARY FIBRE | 4g | VITAMIN C | 20% |
| PROTEIN | 7g | VITAMIN A | 15% |
| | | IRON | 10% |

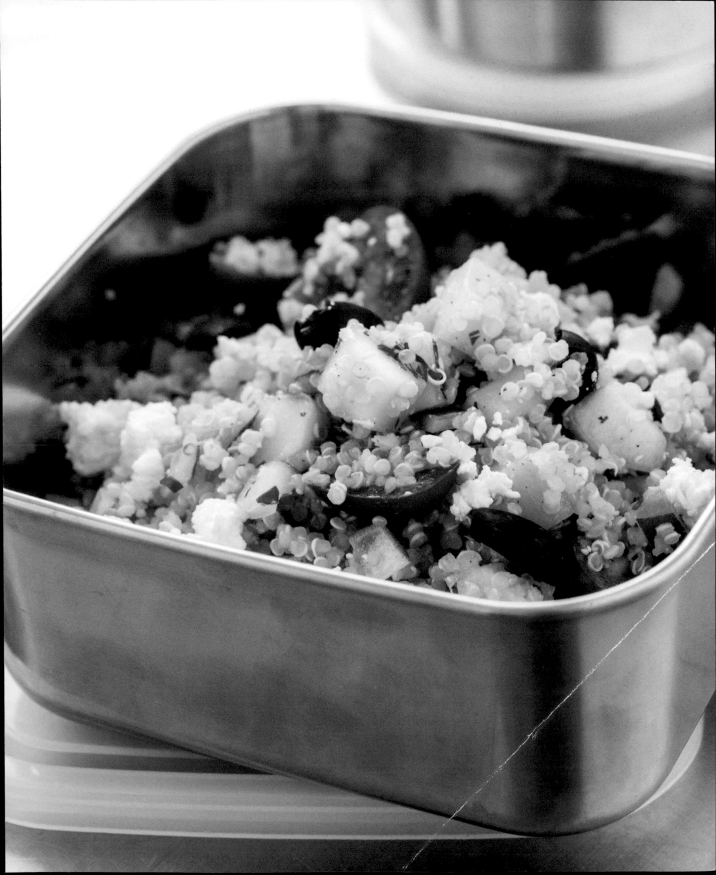

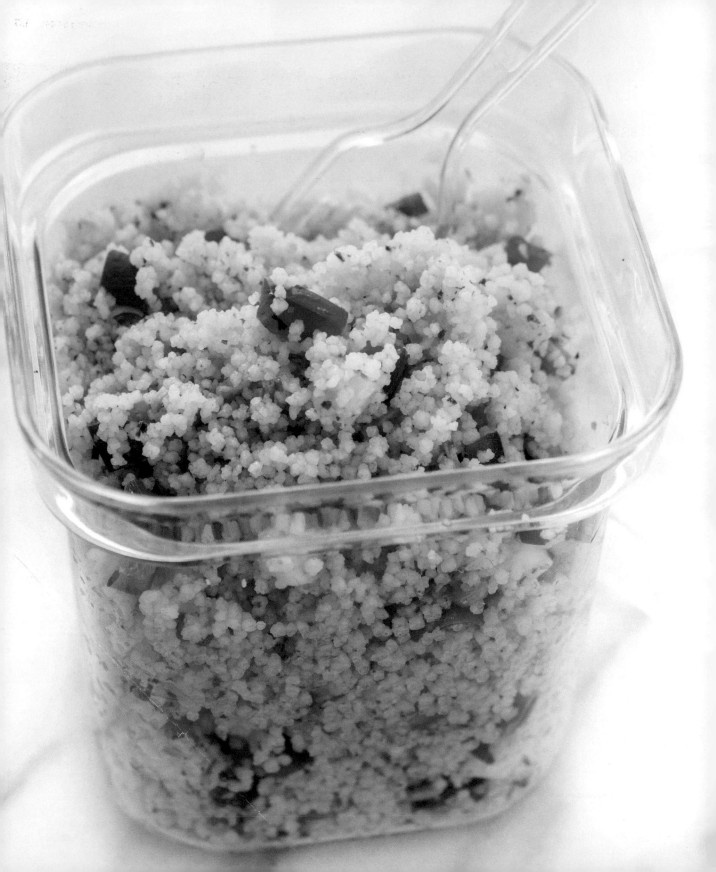

# Super-Simple **Couscous Salad**

This delicious salad, tossed with creamy pesto and tangy feta cheese, is an all-round winner – providing both carbohydrates and protein.

1   Tip the couscous into a large bowl.

2   Boil the water and pour over the couscous. Set aside for 10 minutes or until the water has been absorbed and couscous is fluffy.

3   Once the couscous is cooked, allow it to cool to room temperature.

4   Add the spring onions, pepper, cucumber, feta cheese, pesto sauce, pine nuts, salt, and black pepper, and stir with a fork to combine thoroughly.

5   Allow to chill in the refrigerator for 1–2 hours before serving.

**Make ahead:** Prepare up to 3–5 days ahead, and refrigerate.

If you don't have time to chop your own vegetables, you could always buy a selection of pre-prepared vegetables or try the salad bar at the supermarket.

● **Easy**

**PREP** 5 –10 mins
**COOK** about 18 mins +
            1–2 hours cooling

## SERVES 4

## INGREDIENTS

100g (3½oz) couscous

120ml (4fl oz) water

2 spring onions, sliced

1 small red pepper,
    deseeded and diced

½ medium cucumber,
    deseeded and diced

60g (2oz) reduced fat feta
    cheese, crumbled

1 tbsp pesto

1 tbsp pine nuts

½ tsp salt

¼ tsp freshly ground
    black pepper

To increase the fibre content, use wholewheat couscous or quinoa.

| NUTRITION PER SERVING | | | |
|---|---|---|---|
| ENERGY | 743kJ (177kcal) | FAT | 6.75g |
| CARBOHYDRATES | 20g | CHOLESTEROL | 10mg |
| SUGARS | 2g | SODIUM | 456mg |
| DIETARY FIBRE | 2g | VITAMIN C | 73% |
| PROTEIN | 7g | VITAMIN A | 22% |
| | | IRON | 5% |

# Marinated Greek **Orzo Salad**

This refreshing salad can easily become a nutritious meal in its own right, simply by adding chicken strips or turkey.

● ○ ○ **Easy**

**PREP** 5–10 mins
**COOK** 10 mins + 1 hour
chilling

**SERVES** 6

## INGREDIENTS

160g (5¾oz) orzo pasta

350g (6oz) tinned marinated artichoke hearts, drained with liquid reserved

1 medium tomato, deseeded and diced

1 medium cucumber, deseeded and diced

1 small red onion, diced

150g (5½oz) reduced fat feta cheese, crumbled

30g (1oz) tinned, sliced black olives, drained

15g (½oz) fresh parsley, chopped

Juice of ½ medium lemon (1 tbsp)

½ tsp fresh oregano leaves

½ tsp lemon pepper seasoning

> You can easily adapt this recipe to suit your taste - simply swap the parsley for any other fresh herbs you prefer, such as basil or coriander. Add chicken strips or turkey to increase the protein content.

1   Fill a large pan with water, set over a medium–high heat, and bring to the boil. Add the orzo pasta, and cook for 8–10 minutes or until al dente. Drain and set aside.

2   In a large bowl, combine the cooked pasta, artichoke hearts, tomato, cucumber, red onion, feta cheese, black olives, parsley, lemon juice, oregano, and lemon pepper seasoning. Stir to combine thoroughly and then refrigerate for at least 1 hour.

3   Before serving, drizzle the reserved artichoke marinade over the salad, and toss to coat.

**Make ahead:** Prepare up to 3–5 days ahead, and refrigerate.

| NUTRITION PER SERVING | | | |
|---|---|---|---|
| ENERGY | 840kJ (200kcal) | FAT | 4g |
| CARBOHYDRATES | 29g | CHOLESTEROL | 16.5mg |
| SUGARS | 3.5g | SODIUM | 429mg |
| DIETARY FIBRE | 2.6g | VITAMIN C | 15% |
| PROTEIN | 9.4g | VITAMIN A | 7% |
| | | IRON | 19% |

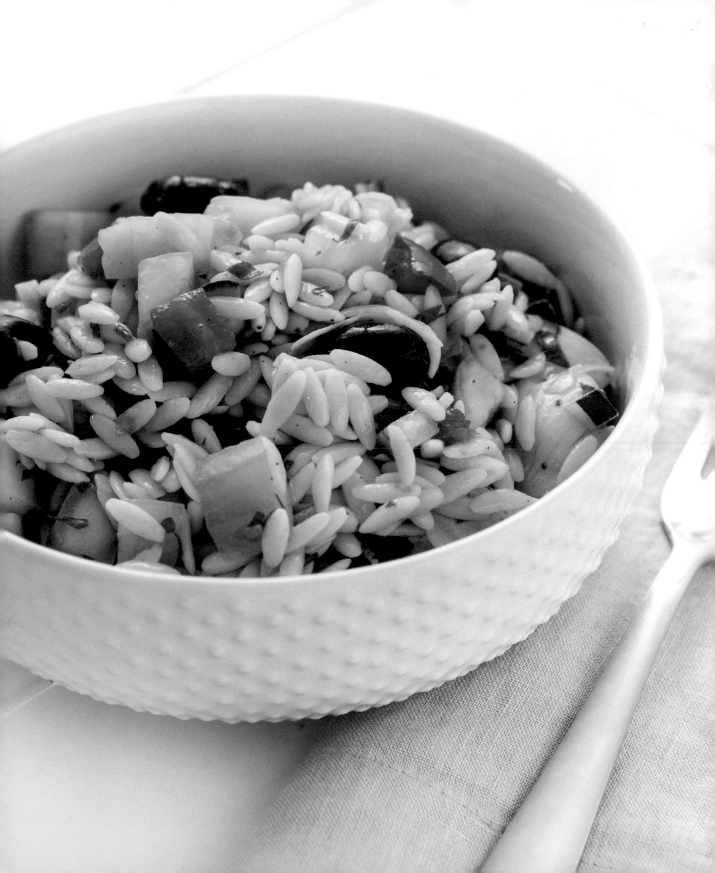

# Chickpea, Tomato, and Mozzarella
## Salad with Pesto

This delicious take on the classic Caprese salad contains protein, fibre, carbs, and electrolytes for recovery.

● ○ ○ **Easy**

**PREP** 5–10 mins

**SERVES** 4

### INGREDIENTS

400g (14oz) canned chickpeas, drained and rinsed

1 tbsp pesto

150g (5½oz) cherry tomatoes, halved

60g (2oz) small fresh mozzarella balls, cut in half

½ tsp salt

¼ tsp freshly ground black pepper

2 tbsp fresh basil, chopped

1 In a medium bowl, gently combine the chickpeas, pesto, cherry tomatoes, mozzarella, salt, and black pepper.

2 Garnish with fresh basil leaves and serve chilled.

**Make ahead:** Prepare up to 3–5 days ahead, and refrigerate.

| NUTRITION PER SERVING | | | |
|---|---|---|---|
| ENERGY | 731kJ (174kcal) | FAT | 6.8g |
| CARBOHYDRATES | 14g | CHOLESTEROL | 12mg |
| SUGARS | 1.4g | SODIUM | 296mg |
| DIETARY FIBRE | 5g | VITAMIN C | 14% |
| PROTEIN | 9g | VITAMIN A | 11% |
| | | IRON | 16% |

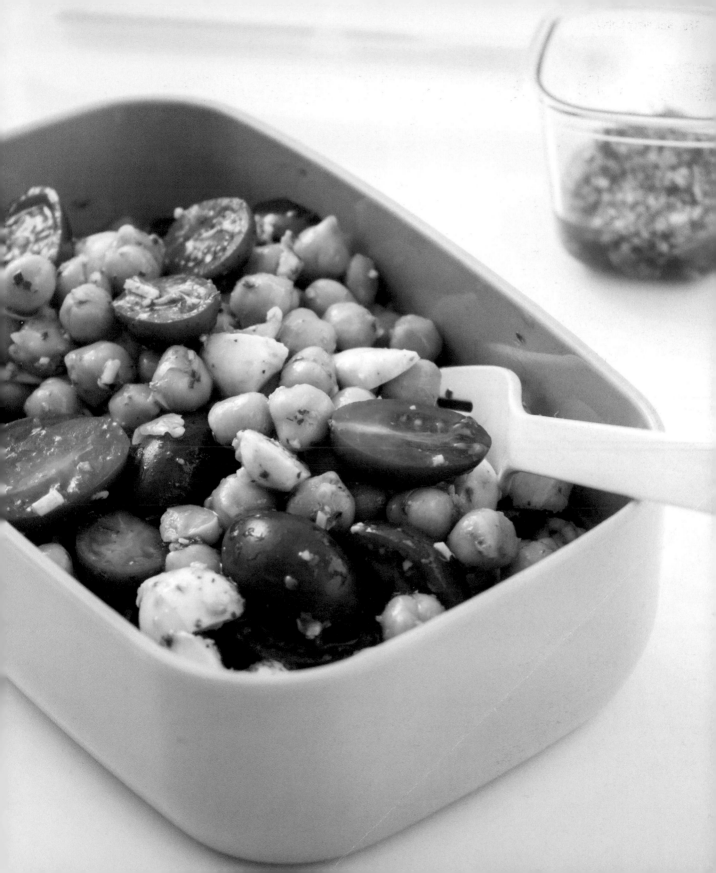

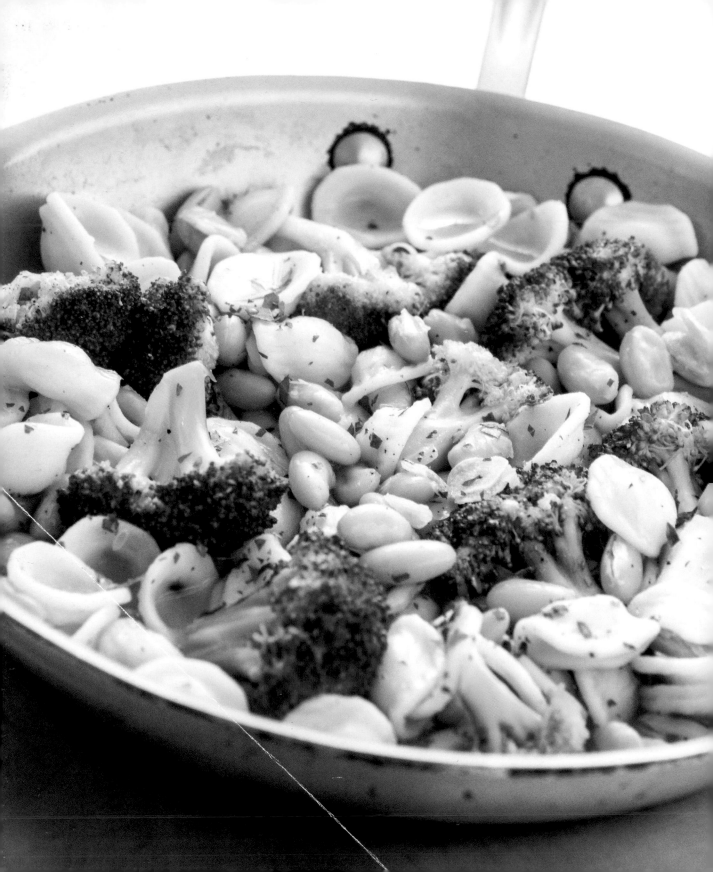

# White Beans and **Broccoli**

This flavoursome and nutritious vegetarian dish contains protein and carbohydrate, and is also high in iron and vitamins A and C.

1 Trim and discard the leaves and tough stem from the broccoli, cut off florets, peel large stems, and cut into 3.75cm (1½in) pieces. Rinse and drain.

2 Heat the oil in a large frying pan over a medium heat. Add the garlic, and cook for 1–2 minutes or until lightly golden.

3 Add the broccoli, chicken stock, crushed chilli flakes, salt, and black pepper, and cook, stirring occasionally, for about 3 minutes.

4 Add the cannellini beans, and cook, stirring occasionally, for about 5 minutes or until the broccoli is just tender and the beans are cooked through.

5 Meanwhile, bring a large pan of water to the boil over a medium–high heat. Add the pasta, and cook for about 8 minutes or until al dente. Drain the pasta, add to the broccoli mixture, and toss to combine.

6 Serve hot.

**Storage:** Refrigerate leftovers for 3–5 days.

## ●● Intermediate

**PREP** 10 mins
**COOK** 15 mins

**SERVES** 6

## INGREDIENTS

675g (1½lb) broccoli

2 tbsp extra-virgin olive oil

2 cloves garlic, minced

80ml (2½fl oz) low-sodium vegetable stock

¼ tsp crushed chilli flakes

½ tsp salt

¼ tsp freshly ground black pepper

800g (28oz) tinned cannellini beans, drained and rinsed

450g (1lb) orecchiette pasta

| NUTRITION PER SERVING | | | |
|---|---|---|---|
| ENERGY | 1,932kJ (460kcal) | FAT | 6g |
| CARBOHYDRATES | 82g | CHOLESTEROL | 0mg |
| SUGARS | 7g | SODIUM | 580mg |
| DIETARY FIBRE | 9g | VITAMIN C | 170% |
| PROTEIN | 23g | VITAMIN A | 150% |
| | | IRON | 30% |

# Basil Penne Pasta with
# Asparagus and Feta

Fresh basil, asparagus, and tomatoes makes this a tasty dish to enjoy while your body recovers.

● **Easy**

**PREP** 10 mins
**COOK** 16 mins

**SERVES** 4

## INGREDIENTS

150g (5½oz) penne pasta

450g (1lb) fresh asparagus, trimmed and cut into 3.75cm (1½in) pieces

1 tbsp extra-virgin olive oil

2 cloves garlic, finely chopped

400g (14oz) tinned cannellini beans, drained and rinsed

225g (8oz) cherry tomatoes, halved

15g (½oz) fresh basil leaves, chopped

1 tbsp fresh lemon juice

½ tsp salt

¼ tsp freshly ground black pepper

175g (6oz) feta cheese, crumbled

To lower the fat content, use reduced fat feta cheese.

1 Fill a large pan with water, set over a medium–high heat, and bring to the boil. Add the pasta, and cook for about 8 minutes or until al dente. During the last 3 minutes of cooking time, add the asparagus.

2 Meanwhile, heat the oil in a large frying pan over a medium heat. Add the garlic, and cook, stirring occasionally, for about 3 minutes.

3 Add the cannellini beans, cherry tomatoes, basil, lemon juice, salt, and black pepper, and toss gently.

4 Stir the cooked pasta and asparagus into the pan, and cook, stirring occasionally, for about 5 minutes or until heated through.

5 Crumble the feta cheese over the top and serve hot.

**Storage:** Refrigerate leftovers for 3–5 days.

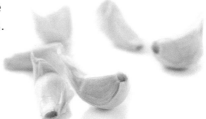

| NUTRITION PER SERVING | | | |
|---|---|---|---|
| ENERGY | 1,781kJ (424kcal) | FAT | 13g |
| CARBOHYDRATES | 56g | CHOLESTEROL | 40mg |
| SUGARS | 9g | SODIUM | 1,050mg |
| DIETARY FIBRE | 9g | VITAMIN C | 30% |
| PROTEIN | 21g | VITAMIN A | 30% |
| | | IRON | 30% |

# Lean Steak and Brown Rice
# **Stir-Fry**

It is good to have a dish that you can make in a hurry, so cook the rice ahead and this stir-fry is on the table in a matter of minutes.

1 In a medium pan over a high heat, bring the water and the brown rice to the boil. Reduce the heat to medium–low, cover, and simmer for 50 minutes. Remove from the heat, and set aside.

2 Meanwhile, trim the fat from the sirloin steak, and cut it into thin strips.

3 Heat the oil in a large frying pan over medium-high heat. Add the garlic, and sauté for 1–2 minutes or until golden.

4 Add the steak, vinegar, salt, black pepper, crushed chilli flakes, and thyme, and cook, stirring occasionally, for about 6 minutes or until the beef is browned.

5 Add the onion and tomato, and cook for 3–5 minutes or until the onions are transparent.

6 Stir in the rice until well combined and serve immediately.

**Storage:** Refrigerate leftovers for 3–5 days.

● **Easy**

**PREP** 10 mins
**COOK** about 1 hour

**SERVES** 6

**INGREDIENTS**

960ml (1¾ pints) water
375 (13oz) brown rice
450g (1lb) sirloin steak
2 tbsp extra-virgin olive oil
1 clove garlic, finely chopped
½ tsp red wine vinegar
½ tsp salt
¼ tsp freshly ground
   black pepper
¼ tsp crushed chilli flakes
¼ tsp fresh thyme leaves
1 small sweet onion, sliced
1 medium tomato, diced

| NUTRITION PER SERVING | | | |
|---|---|---|---|
| ENERGY | 1,848kJ (440kcal) | FAT | 14g |
| CARBOHYDRATES | 50g | CHOLESTEROL | 55mg |
| SUGARS | 2g | SODIUM | 150mg |
| DIETARY FIBRE | 3g | VITAMIN C | 8% |
| PROTEIN | 27g | VITAMIN A | 6% |
| | | IRON | 15% |

To make this recipe vegetarian, use 450g (1lb) extra-firm tofu, cut into 1cm (½in) cubes. Add the tofu at the same time as you would the steak and continue with the recipe.

# Courgette Pizza **Casserole**

This family-size casserole is packed full of vegetables. It's quick and easy to prepare, and tastes delicious - just like a classic pizza!

● ● ●  **Easy**

**PREP** 2 mins
**COOK** 1 hour, 5 mins

**SERVES** 8

## INGREDIENTS

6 medium courgettes, grated

½ tsp salt

2 large eggs

½ tsp freshly ground
   black pepper

½ tsp crushed chilli flakes

50g (1¾oz) Parmesan
   cheese, grated

225g (8oz) low-fat mozzarella
   cheese, grated

115g (4oz) Cheddar
   cheese, grated

450g (1lb) lean minced beef

1 small yellow onion, diced

425g (15oz) jar tomato sauce

1 medium green pepper,
   deseeded and diced

To make this recipe vegetarian, replace the minced beef with any meat alternatives, such as tofu.

1  Preheat the oven to 200°C (400°F/gas 6). Lightly grease a 23 × 33cm (9 × 13in) baking dish with cooking spray.

2  Strain the grated courgette in a sieve, sprinkle with salt, and set aside for 10 minutes. Squeeze out the excess moisture.

3  In the prepared dish, combine the courgette, eggs, black pepper, crushed chilli flakes, Parmesan, and half of the mozzarella and Cheddar cheeses. Press the mixture into the bottom of the dish.

4  Bake uncovered for 20 minutes.

5  Meanwhile, in a medium frying pan over a medium heat, cook the beef and onion for 5–10 minutes or until the meat is no longer pink. Drain off any fat.

6  Add the tomato sauce, stir to combine, and spoon the sauce over the courgette mixture. Sprinkle with the remaining mozzarella and Cheddar cheeses, and add the green pepper. Bake for 20 minutes or until heated through.

7  Allow to rest for 8–10 minutes before serving.

**Make ahead and freeze:** Prepare up to the end of step 3 up to 6 days ahead. Freeze after step 6 for up to 2 months. Thaw in the refrigerator for 1 or 2 days before baking.

| NUTRITION PER SERVING | | | |
|---|---|---|---|
| ENERGY | 1,050kJ (250kcal) | FAT | 10g |
| CARBOHYDRATES | 10g | CHOLESTEROL | 105mg |
| SUGARS | 4g | SODIUM | 910mg |
| DIETARY FIBRE | 3g | VITAMIN C | 90% |
| PROTEIN | 31g | VITAMIN A | 25% |
| | | IRON | 15% |

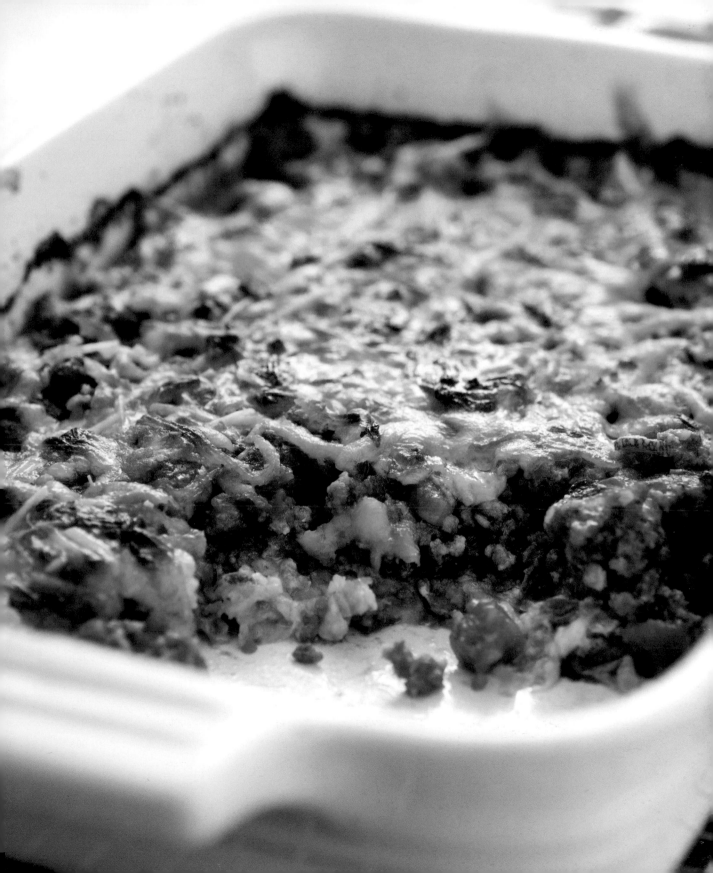

# Chicken with Orzo **Pasta**

This delicious and simple chicken dish – with fresh spinach, nutty Parmesan cheese, and a little heat from the crushed chillies – is also a good source of protein, carbs, and iron.

● Easy

**PREP** 10 mins
**COOK** about 20 mins

**SERVES** 4

**INGREDIENTS**

115g (4oz) orzo pasta

1 tbsp extra-virgin olive oil

2 cloves garlic, finely chopped

¼ tsp crushed chilli flakes

450g (8oz) boneless, skinless chicken breasts, cut into 2.5cm (1in) cubes

½ tsp salt

½ tsp freshly ground black pepper

1 tbsp fresh parsley, chopped

60g (2oz) fresh baby spinach

50g (1¾oz) Parmesan cheese

1  Fill a large pan with water, set over a medium–high heat, and bring to the boil. Add the pasta, and cook for 8–10 minutes or until al dente. Drain.

2  Heat the oil in a medium frying pan over a medium-high heat. Add the garlic and crushed chilli flakes, and cook for about 1 minute or until the garlic is lightly golden.

3  Stir in the chicken, salt, and black pepper, and cook for 2–5 minutes or until lightly browned and the chicken is cooked through.

4  Reduce the heat to medium, and mix in the parsley and the cooked pasta. Add the baby spinach, and continue cooking, stirring occasionally, for about 5 minutes or until the spinach is wilted.

5  Grate the Parmesan, stir it in, and serve the dish hot.

**Storage:** Refrigerate leftovers for 3–5 days.

For a vegetarian version, use 450g (1lb) extra-firm tofu, cut into 1cm (½in) cubes. Add the tofu at the same time as the chicken would have been added, and continue the recipe as directed above.

| NUTRITION PER SERVING | | | |
|---|---|---|---|
| ENERGY | 1,624kJ (387kcal) | FAT | 10.34g |
| CARBOHYDRATES | 39g | CHOLESTEROL | 80mg |
| SUGARS | 2g | SODIUM | 600mg |
| DIETARY FIBRE | 2g | VITAMIN C | 8% |
| PROTEIN | 35g | VITAMIN A | 15% |
| | | IRON | 15% |

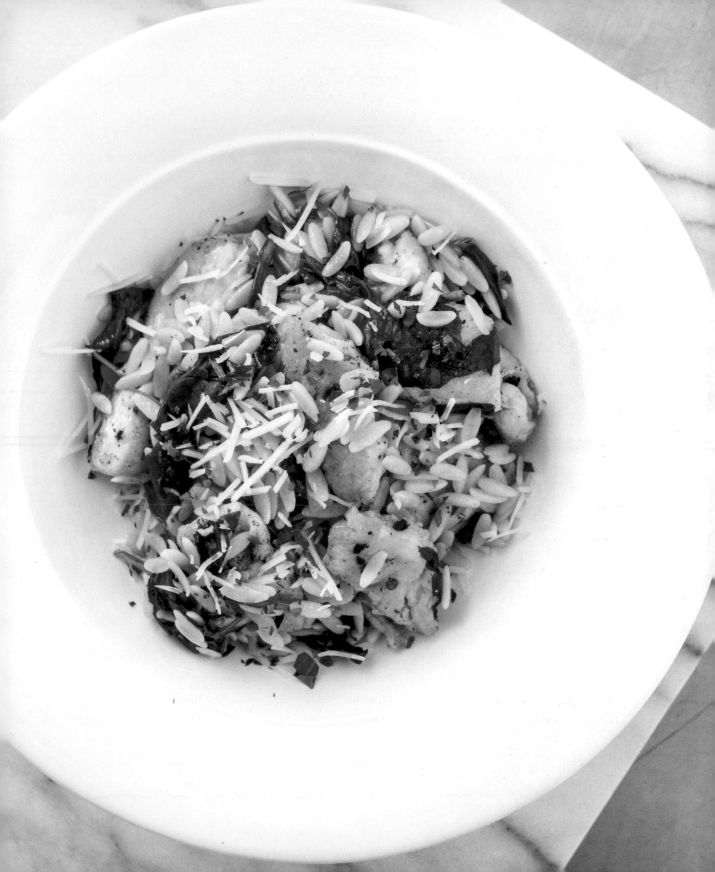

# Slow-Cooker **Beef and Cabbage**

A high energy meal with plenty of protein and carbohydrate to help your body recover, as well as being an excellent source of vitamins A and C.

● ● ○ **Intermediate**

**PREP** 15 mins
**COOK** 6 hours

**SERVES** 8

## INGREDIENTS

1.5kg (3lb 3oz) beef brisket

1 tsp salt

10g (¼oz) pickling spice

1 small cabbage, cut into wedges

4 medium carrots, peeled and cut into 5cm (2in) pieces

1 medium yellow onion, cut into wedges

18 Anya or pink fir apple potatoes

120ml (4fl oz) water

**1** Cut the beef so that it fits into a 4.75–5.5-litre (8¼–9½-pint) slow cooker. Evenly sprinkle the spices over the brisket, and rub in with your fingers.

**2** Add the cabbage, carrots, yellow onion, and potatoes to the slow cooker.

**3** Pour the water over the vegetables, and sit the brisket on top.

**4** Cover and cook on high for 6 hours or until the meat is fork-tender.

**5** Remove the brisket from the slow cooker, slice, and serve with the vegetables.

**Make ahead:** Refrigerate leftovers 3–5 days.

To lower the fat in this recipe, trim off any excess fat from the beef brisket before cooking. Make your own pickling spice by combining mustard seeds, allspice, coriander seeds, cloves, ginger, red pepper flakes, a bay leaf and cinnamon.

| NUTRITION PER SERVING | | | |
|---|---|---|---|
| ENERGY | 2,730kJ (650kcal) | FAT | 26g |
| CARBOHYDRATES | 70g | CHOLESTEROL | 90mg |
| SUGARS | 9g | SODIUM | 2,150mg |
| DIETARY FIBRE | 9g | VITAMIN C | 200% |
| PROTEIN | 34g | VITAMIN A | 100% |
| | | IRON | 30% |

# Spaghetti with **Meat Sauce**

This classic, easy-to-make dish provides carbohydrate and protein that will help you recover after a hard workout or competition.

1   In a large pan over a medium–high heat, combine the oil, beef, onion, garlic, and green pepper. Cook, stirring occasionally, for about 5 minutes or until the meat is browned and vegetables are tender. Drain off any fat.

2   Stir in the chopped tomatoes, passata, and tomato purée. Season with oregano, basil, salt, and black pepper. Simmer the sauce, stirring occasionally, for 1 hour.

3   When the sauce is about 10 minutes from being done, fill a large pan with water, and set over a medium–high heat. Bring water to the boil and cook the spaghetti, stirring occasionally, for about 8 minutes or until al dente.

4   Evenly divide the spaghetti and sauce between 8 plates or bowls, and serve immediately.

**Make ahead:** Prepare the meat sauce up to 3–5 days ahead and refrigerate, or freeze for up to 2 months.

To cook this in a slow cooker, complete step 1 as above and then add all the ingredients (except for the pasta) to a 4.75-litre (8¼-pint) slow cooker. Cover and cook on low for 6–8 hours. Cook the pasta when the sauce is just about finished cooking, and serve as above.

● ○ ○   **Easy**

**PREP** 15 mins
**COOK** 1 hour, 15 mins

**SERVES** 8

### INGREDIENTS

450g (1lb) lean minced beef

1 tbsp olive oil

1 small yellow onion, chopped

4 cloves garlic, finely chopped

1 small green pepper, deseeded and diced

800g (28oz) tinned chopped tomatoes, with juice

450g (1lb) tomato passata

175g (6oz) tomato purée

2 tsp dried oregano

2 tsp dried basil

1 tsp salt

½ tsp freshly ground black pepper

450g (1lb) spaghetti

| NUTRITION PER SERVING | | | |
|---|---|---|---|
| ENERGY | 1,664kJ (396kcal) | FAT | 8.8g |
| CARBOHYDRATES | 55g | CHOLESTEROL | 35mg |
| SUGARS | 10g | SODIUM | 860mg |
| DIETARY FIBRE | 4g | VITAMIN C | 60% |
| PROTEIN | 21g | VITAMIN A | 20% |
| | | IRON | 20% |

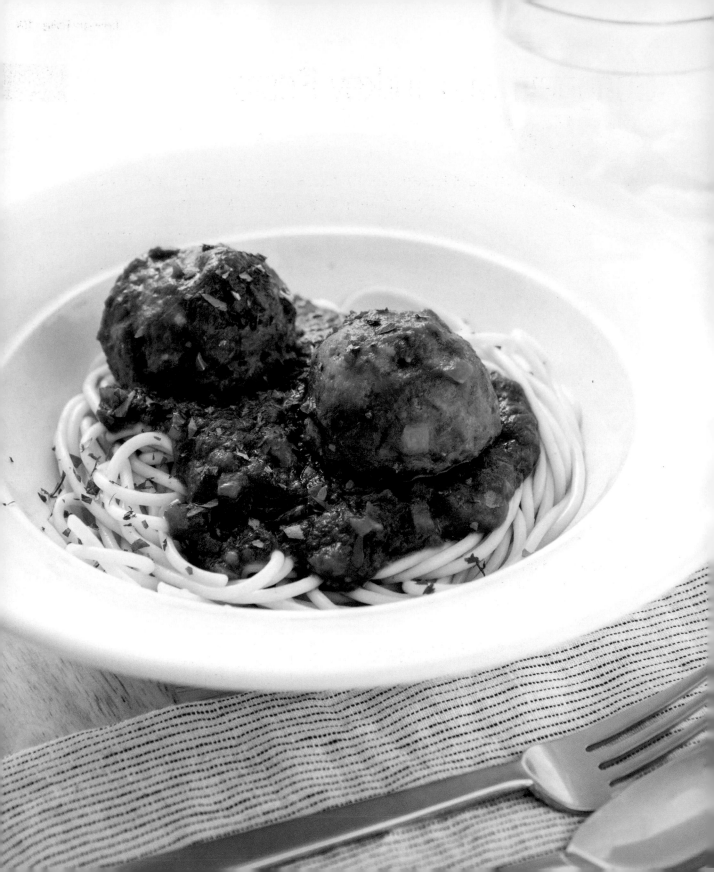

# Spaghetti with Turkey Pesto
# Meatballs

Make a switch from beef meatballs to these lower-fat turkey ones so that this carb-loaded meal becomes full of lean protein, too.

1   Spread 240ml (8fl oz) of the tomato pasta sauce in the bottom of a medium, heavy frying pan.

2   In a medium bowl, combine the turkey, breadcrumbs, pesto, egg white, garlic, and salt. Using your hands, form the mixture into 4 medium meatballs.

3   Place the meatballs in a single layer in the pan, and spoon the remaining pasta sauce over the top.

4   Set the pan over a medium heat, and bring it to a simmer. Cover, reduce the heat to medium low, and simmer, stirring occasionally, for 25–30 minutes or until the meatballs are cooked through.

5   Meanwhile, fill a large pan with water, and set over a medium–high heat. Bring the water to the boil, add the spaghetti, and cook for about 10 minutes or until just tender but still firm to the bite.

6   Drain the pasta and divide between 2 bowls. Top with meatballs and sauce, and serve hot.

**Make ahead and freeze:** Prepare up to the end of step 3 up to 3 days ahead. Freeze after step 3 for up to 2 months. Thaw in the refrigerator for 4 or 5 hours before baking.

● ●   **Intermediate**

**PREP** 15–20 mins
**COOK** about 40 mins

**SERVES** 2

**INGREDIENTS**

520g (1lb 3oz) jar chunky
   tomato pasta sauce
225g (8oz) minced turkey
30g (1oz) dried breadcrumbs
1 tbsp pesto
1 large egg white
1 tsp garlic, finely chopped
¼ tsp salt
225g (8oz) spaghetti

| NUTRITION PER SERVING | | | |
|---|---|---|---|
| ENERGY | 294kJ (700kcal) | FAT | 19.6g |
| CARBOHYDRATES | 95g | CHOLESTEROL | 70mg |
| SUGARS | 8.6g | SODIUM | 1,004mg |
| DIETARY FIBRE | 7.7g | VITAMIN C | 27% |
| PROTEIN | 46g | VITAMIN A | 12% |
| | | IRON | 34% |

To lower the fat of the recipe even further, use the turkey breast mince only. Minced turkey can often include other parts of the turkey, such as the skin, which is higher in fat.

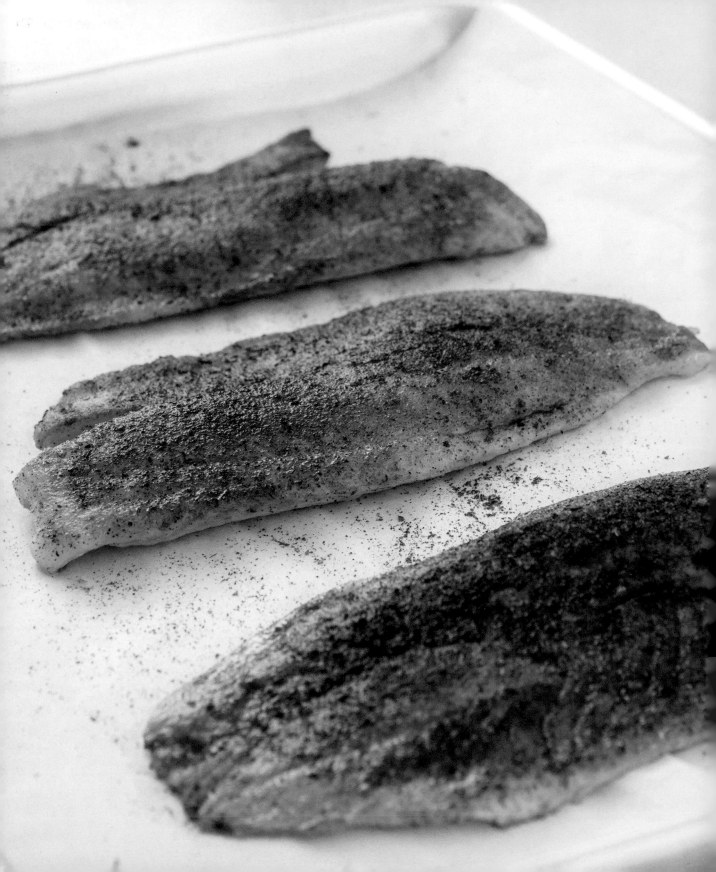

# Blackened **Hake**

Naturally low in fat, white fish easily takes on flavours. Here, we rub it with spice and blacken it to perfection. Serve with baked potato wedges or rice and salad for a balanced recovery meal.

1 Preheat the oven to 220°C (425°F/gas 7). Line a baking tray with baking parchment.

2 In a small bowl, combine the paprika, salt, onion powder, black pepper, cayenne, thyme, oregano, and garlic powder.

3 Rinse and pat dry the hake fillets, brush with the oil, and completely coat with the seasoning mixture. Place the hake on the prepared baking tray and spray lightly with cooking spray.

4 Bake the hake for 15–20 minutes or until golden brown and cooked through.

5 Serve immediately.

**Storage:** Refrigerate leftovers for 3–5 days.

To make this dish vegetarian, substitute the hake with 4 x 115g (4oz) portions of extra-firm tofu, drained, and coated with the seasoning as for the fish. Cook in the same way.

● ○ ○   **Easy**

**PREP** 8 mins
**COOK** 15–20 mins

**SERVES** 4

**INGREDIENTS**

3 tbsp paprika

1 tsp salt

1 tbsp onion powder

1 tsp freshly ground
    black pepper

½ tsp cayenne pepper

1 tsp dried thyme

1 tsp dried oregano

1 tsp garlic powder

450g (1lb) hake fillets

1 tbsp extra-virgin olive oil

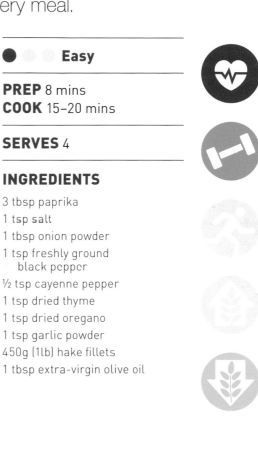

Reserve any leftover seasoning – that didn't come into contact with the fish – and use it when cooking beef, chicken, or even pork.

### NUTRITION PER SERVING

| | | | |
|---|---|---|---|
| ENERGY | 630kJ (150 kcal) | FAT | 6g |
| CARBOHYDRATES | 3g | CHOLESTEROL | 55mg |
| SUGARS | 0g | SODIUM | 640mg |
| DIETARY FIBRE | 2g | VITAMIN C | 6% |
| PROTEIN | 23g | VITAMIN A | 50% |
| | | IRON | 10% |

# Garlic and Butter **Prawns**

This high-protein dish, thanks to the prawns, features zesty garlic, spice from black pepper and crushed chilli flakes, and a splash of citrus.

● ● ○  **Intermediate**

**PREP** 10 mins
**COOK** 5 mins

**SERVES** 4

## INGREDIENTS

1 tbsp salted butter

1 tbsp extra-virgin olive oil

4 cloves garlic, sliced

¼ tsp crushed red pepper flakes

450g (1lb) prawns, shelled and deveined

120ml (4fl oz) white wine

2 tbsp fresh parsley, chopped

¼ tsp freshly cracked black pepper

Juice of ½ medium lemon (1 tbsp)

1 In a large frying pan over a medium heat, heat the butter and oil together until the butter is melted. Add the garlic and crushed chilli flakes, and sauté for 1 minute or until the garlic begins to lightly brown.

2 Add the prawns and the white wine, increase the heat to high, and cook for 2–3 minutes. Flip over the prawns, and cook for a further minute. Remove the pan from the heat.

3 Sprinkle the parsley and black pepper over the prawns, and drizzle the lemon juice over the top. Toss to combine, and serve hot.

**Storage:** Refrigerate leftovers for 2–3 days.

This is a great recipe to serve as a main dish with a number of different sides. To turn it into an easy meal, serve with pasta.

| NUTRITION PER SERVING | | | |
|---|---|---|---|
| ENERGY | 809kJ (193kcal) | FAT | 6.5g |
| CARBOHYDRATES | 2g | CHOLESTEROL | 235mg |
| SUGARS | 0g | SODIUM | 300mg |
| DIETARY FIBRE | 0g | VITAMIN C | 8% |
| PROTEIN | 24g | VITAMIN A | 10% |
| | | IRON | 20% |

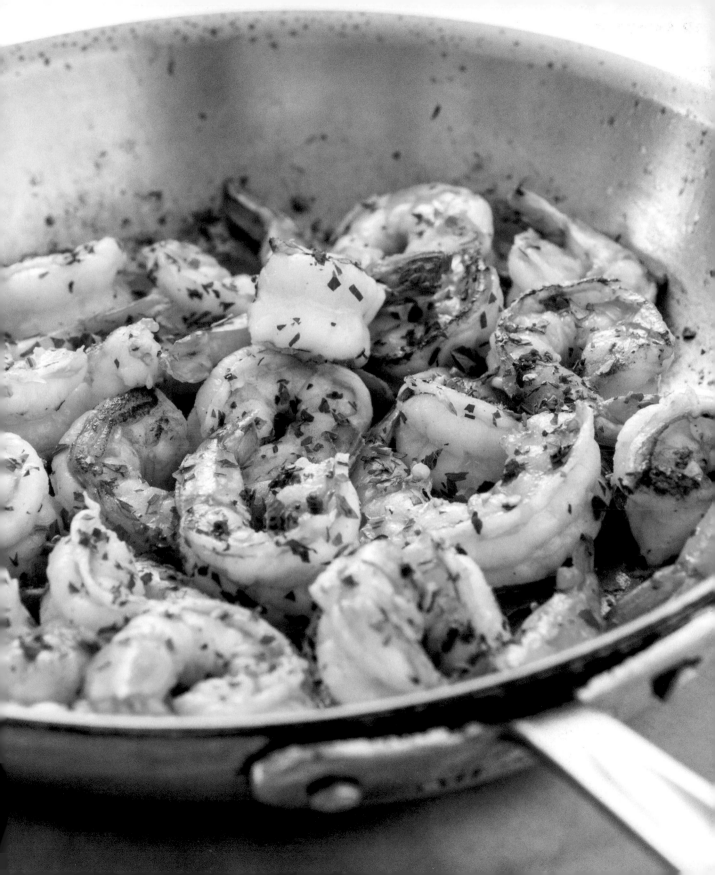

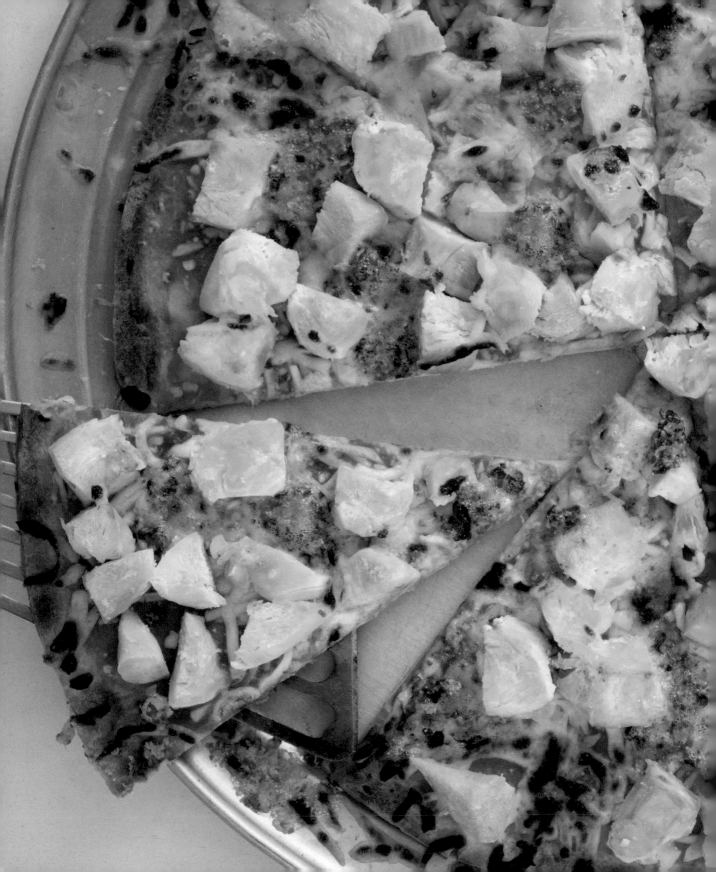

# Buffalo Chicken **Pizza**

You can vary the toppings of this pizza to suit your tastes. Try using seafood, lean ham, pineapple, and any vegetables you enjoy.

**1**  Preheat the oven to 180°C (350°F/gas 4).

**2**  Place the pizza base on a baking stone or baking tray. Spread the hot sauce over the base, and layer the chicken, mozzarella, and blue cheeses on top.

**3**  Bake on the baking stone or tray for 20–25 minutes or until the cheese has melted and is bubbly.

**Make ahead and freeze:** Prepare up to the end of step 2 up to 3 days ahead. Freeze after step 3 for up to 2 months. Bake from frozen.

● ○ ○   **Easy**

**PREP** 5 mins
**COOK** 25 mins

**SERVES** 8

## INGREDIENTS

450g (1lb) plain pizza base

120ml (4fl oz) jar spicy tomato pasta sauce

300g (10oz) cooked chicken breast, diced

115g (4oz) reduced-fat mozzarella cheese, grated

60g (2oz) blue cheese, crumbled

| NUTRITION PER SERVING | | | |
|---|---|---|---|
| ENERGY | 1,134kJ (270 kcal) | FAT | 8g |
| CARBOHYDRATES | 29g | CHOLESTEROL | 30mg |
| SUGARS | 1g | SODIUM | 1,090mg |
| DIETARY FIBRE | 2g | VITAMIN C | 0% |
| PROTEIN | 18g | VITAMIN A | 4% |
| | | IRON | 10% |

To make this recipe gluten free, choose a gluten-free pizza base. To make it vegetarian, substitute firm tofu, crumbled, or seitan for the chicken breast.

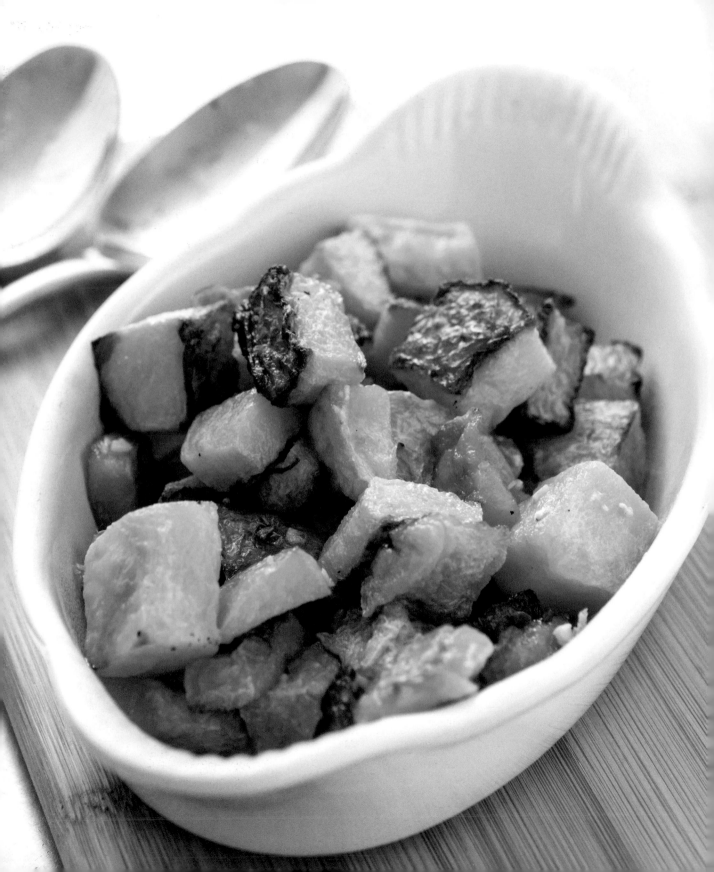

# Roasted **Butternut Squash**

Butternut squash, high in vitamin A, is simply seasoned and oven-roasted in this dish. A savoury side to warm you up on a cold day.

1  Preheat the oven to 200°C (400°F/gas 6).

2  In a large bowl, toss the butternut squash with the oil, garlic, salt, and black pepper. Spread the squash out onto a baking tray.

3  Roast for about 25–30 minutes or until the squash is tender and lightly browned.

4  Serve immediately.

**Storage:** Refrigerate leftovers for 3–5 days.

● ○ ○  **Easy**

**PREP** 15 mins
**COOK** 25–30 mins

**SERVES** 4

**INGREDIENTS**

1 butternut squash (1–1.5kg; 2¼–3¼lb), peeled, deseeded, and cut into 2.5cm (1in) cubes

1 tbsp extra-virgin olive oil

2 cloves garlic, finely chopped

1 tsp salt

½ tsp freshly ground black pepper

For a quick squash soup, blend all cooked ingredients for 2 or 3 minutes with 480ml (15½fl oz) of low-fat milk and 2 tablespoons of honey. Add the blended butternut squash mixture to a medium pan over a medium–low heat, and cook, stirring occasionally, for about 5 minutes or until heated through. Adjust seasoning and serve hot.

| NUTRITION PER SERVING | | | |
|---|---|---|---|
| ENERGY | 938kJ (223kcal) | FAT | 3.3g |
| CARBOHYDRATES | 34g | CHOLESTEROL | 0mg |
| SUGARS | 6g | SODIUM | 590mg |
| DIETARY FIBRE | 6g | VITAMIN C | 100% |
| PROTEIN | 3g | VITAMIN A | 610% |
| | | IRON | 10% |

# Reduced-Fat **Creamed Spinach**

This comfort-food side dish has all the flavour of traditional creamed spinach but is much lower in fat and calories – hooray!

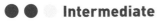

● ● ⬤ **Intermediate**

**PREP** 5–10 mins
**COOK** about 12 mins

**SERVES** 6

## INGREDIENTS

1 tbsp extra-virgin
   olive oil, plus 2 tsp

900g (2lb) fresh baby spinach

1 tsp salt

½ tsp freshly ground
   black pepper

⅛ tsp cayenne pepper

⅛ tsp ground nutmeg

2 tbsp minced shallots

180ml (6fl oz) whole milk

1 tsp freshly grated lemon zest

2 tbsp grated Parmesan cheese

1 Heat the 2 teaspoons of oil in a large pan over a medium heat. Add the baby spinach, cover, and cook for about 1 minute. Uncover, and stir until all the leaves are wilted.

2 Drain the spinach in a sieve and transfer to a kitchen-paper-lined plate. When the spinach is cool enough to handle, squeeze out as much liquid as possible, transfer it to a chopping board, and roughly chop.

3 In a small bowl, combine the salt, black pepper, cayenne pepper, and nutmeg.

4 Heat the remaining oil in the same large pan over a medium heat. Add the shallots, stir, and cook for about 3–4 minutes or until just golden brown.

5 Stir in the seasoning mixture and whole milk, and cook for about 5 minutes or until the milk is reduced by about half.

6 Stir in the lemon zest.

7 Reduce the heat to low, add the spinach, and cook, stirring, for about 2 minutes or until the spinach is heated through and coated with the sauce.

8 Stir in the Parmesan and serve immediately.

**Storage:** Refrigerate leftovers for 3–5 days.

To lower the fat content, replace whole milk with semi-skimmed milk.

| NUTRITION PER SERVING | | | |
|---|---|---|---|
| ENERGY | 500kJ (120kcal) | FAT | 5g |
| CARBOHYDRATES | 18g | CHOLESTEROL | 5mg |
| SUGARS | 2g | SODIUM | 670mg |
| DIETARY FIBRE | 7g | VITAMIN C | 35% |
| PROTEIN | 5g | VITAMIN A | 110% |
| | | IRON | 25% |

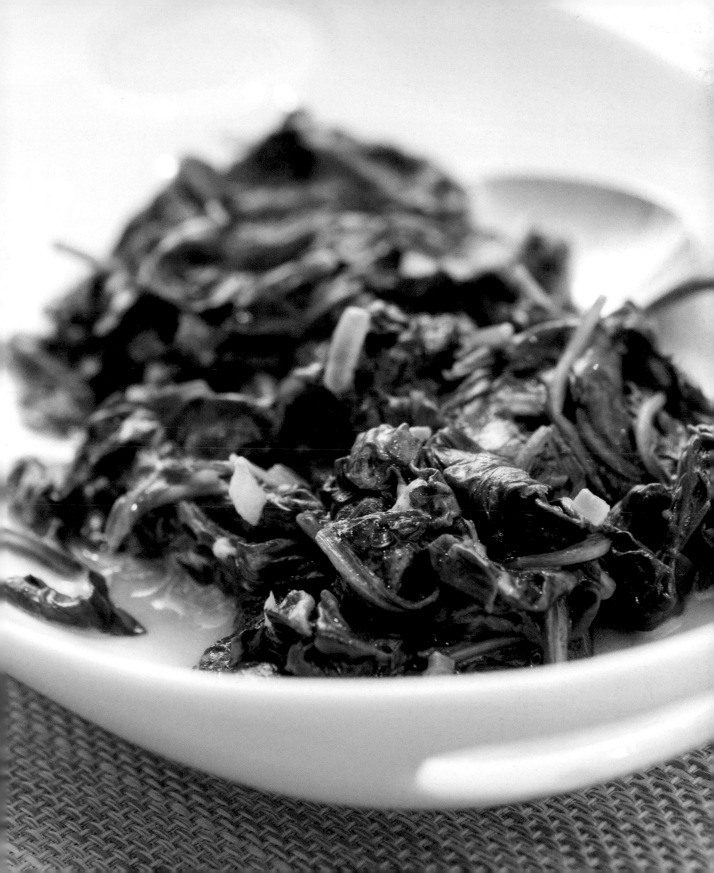

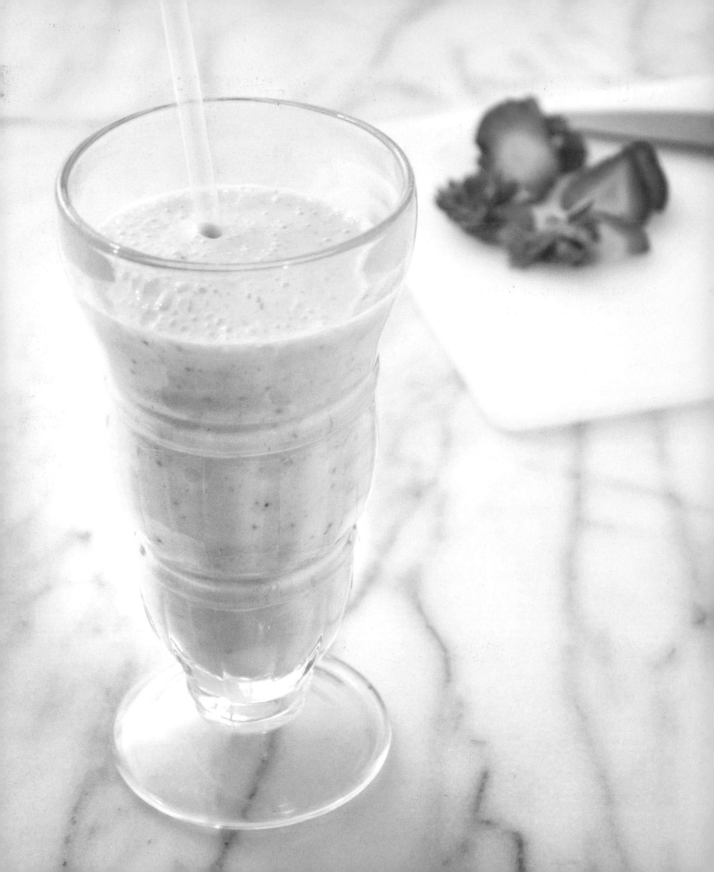

# Strawberry Shortcake **Milkshake**

With plenty of carbohydrate and 14 grams of protein per serving, this super-powered smoothie is high in vitamin C and ideal for recovery.

1  In a blender, blend the yoghurt, skimmed milk, strawberries, rolled oats, sugar, and vanilla extract for about 3 minutes or until smooth.

2  Serve immediately.

**Storage:** Refrigerate leftovers in a sealed cup, and stir when ready to drink.

● ○ ○  **Easy**

**PREP** 5 mins

**SERVES** 3

### INGREDIENTS

480ml (16fl oz) low-fat plain yoghurt

480ml (16fl oz) skimmed milk

300g (10oz) fresh or frozen strawberries

25g (scant 1oz) rolled oats

2 tbsp granulated sugar

1 tsp vanilla extract

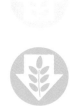

| NUTRITION PER SERVING | | | | |
|---|---|---|---|---|
| ENERGY | 1,121kJ (267kcal) | FAT | 4.5g |
| CARBOHYDRATES | 39g | CHOLESTEROL | 16mg |
| SUGARS | 34g | SODIUM | 194mg |
| DIETARY FIBRE | 2.7g | VITAMIN C | 76% |
| PROTEIN | 14g | VITAMIN A | 5% |
| | | IRON | 9% |

# Meal **Plans**

In this appendix, we share meal plans, one for endurance athletes and one for strength athletes. Both have been prepared for an athlete who weighs 82kg (12 stone 12lb), and workout/competition times for this athlete are in the afternoon. Use these menus as a guideline for how you could set up your own so you're sure to consume enough nutrition and meet your body's needs.

## ENDURANCE ATHLETES

See Determining Your Energy Requirements (page 16) for guidance in adapting this meal plan to your situation.

Nutrition based on an 82kg (12 stone 12lb) athlete.

**DAILY NUTRITION**

**Energy:** 12,500kJ (3,000kcal)

**Fat:** 80–90g

**Carbohydrates:** 500–600g

**Protein:** 90–110g

| Meal/Snack | Timing | Menu Item | Nutrition |
|---|---|---|---|
| Breakfast | | 1 serving Super-Quick Breakfast Burritos<br>240ml (8fl oz) low-fat milk<br>1 medium banana<br>240ml (8fl oz) 100% fruit juice | 2,114kJ (507kcal)<br>11g fat<br>84g carbohydrates<br>22g protein |
| Morning snack | | 160g (5¾oz) strawberries<br>150g (5½oz) blueberries<br>1 serving Low-Fat Banana Bread<br>240ml (8fl oz) 100% fruit juice | 1,518kJ (364kcal)<br>4g fat<br>81g carbohydrates<br>7g protein |
| Lunch | 3 or 4 hours before training/competition | 1 serving Wholemeal Turkey and Veggie Pitta Sandwich<br>1 serving Quick Tortellini Salad<br>1 medium apple<br>240ml (8fl oz) low-fat chocolate milk<br>240ml (8fl oz) 100% fruit juice | 3,374kJ (809kcal)<br>21g fat<br>135g carbohydrates<br>31g protein |
| Afternoon snack | 1 hour before training/competition | 10 hard pretzels<br>85g (3oz) grapes | 1,214kJ (289kcal)<br>2g fat<br>64g carbohydrates<br>7g protein |
| Training/competition | During training/competition | 1 serving Quick and Easy Energy Bars<br>1 serving Mango Cooler | 1,638kJ (390kcal)<br>12g fat<br>71g carbohydrates<br>4g protein |
| Dinner | 30 minutes to 1 hour after training/competition | 1 serving Slow Cooker Pot Roast<br>185g (6½oz) white rice<br>85g (3oz) mixed vegetables<br>240ml (8fl oz) 100% fruit juice | 2,843kJ (677kcal)<br>18g fat<br>81g carbohydrates<br>32g protein |
| Evening snack | | 150g (5½oz) orange sorbet | 1092kJ (260kcal)<br>4g fat<br>54g carbohydrates<br>2g protein |

**TOTAL NUTRITIONAL BREAKDOWN**

**Energy:** 13,843kJ (3,296 kcal)

**Fat:** 72g

**Carbohydrates:** 498g

**Protein:** 105g

## ADAPTING PLANS

To adjust the sample menus, determine your caloric needs, and add or subtract calories (and the associated menu items) to fit your needs. Make substitutions for snacks or main dishes as needed.

If you have a workout/competition in the morning, rearrange the sample menu as appropriate to the time when you have your workout/competition and use the timing guidelines as recommended.

### STRENGTH ATHLETES

See Determining Your Energy Requirements (page 16) for guidance in adapting this meal plan to your situation.

Nutrition based on an 82kg (12 stone 12lb) athlete.

**DAILY NUTRITION**

**Energy:** 12,500kJ (3,000kcal)

**Fat:** 70–80g

**Carbohydrates:** 400–500g

**Protein:** 120–140g

| Meal/Snack | Timing | Menu Item | Nutrition |
|---|---|---|---|
| Breakfast | | 240ml (8fl oz) cooked oatmeal (add 2 tbsp brown sugar, 1 tbsp sliced almonds, and 30g (1oz) fresh blueberries)<br>240ml (8fl oz) low-fat milk<br>1 medium banana | 1,676kJ (399kcal)<br>16g fat<br>66g carbohydrates<br>13g protein |
| Morning snack | | 240ml (8fl oz) low-fat yogurt<br>1 Sweet and Salty Peanut Bar<br>85g (3oz) grapes | 2,200kJ (524kcal)<br>15g fat<br>101g carbohydrates<br>23g protein |
| Lunch | 3 or 4 hours before training/competition | 1 serving Prawn and Spinach Pasta<br>1 medium apple<br>240ml (8fl oz) 100% fruit juice | 3,217kJ (766kcal)<br>11g fat<br>106g carbohydrates<br>39g protein |
| Afternoon snack | 1 hour before training/competition | 1 serving Acai Punch<br>1 medium apple | 710kJ (169kcal)<br>0g fat<br>42g carbohydrates<br>0g protein |
| Training/competition | During training/competition | 1 serving Blueberry Madness Bars<br>1 serving Blackberry Cooler | 1,554kJ (370kcal)<br>16g fat<br>52g carbohydrates<br>4g protein |
| Dinner | 30 minutes to 1 hour after training/competition | 1 serving Beef, Broccoli, and Sweet Potato Stir-Fry<br>275g (11oz) white rice<br>240ml (8fl oz) 100% fruit juice | 3,343kJ (796kcal)<br>19g fat<br>103g carbohydrates<br>34g protein |
| Evening snack | | 1 serving Lavender Lemonade Relaxer<br>160g (5¾oz) sliced strawberries with 4 tbsp low-fat whipped topping or sweetened whipped cream | 1,029kJ (245kcal)<br>2g fat<br>71g carbohydrate<br>1g protein |

**TOTAL NUTRITIONAL BREAKDOWN**

**Energy:** 13,730kJ (3,269kcal)

**Fat:** 79g

**Carbohydrates:** 541g

**Protein:** 118g

# Common **Conversions**

All recipes in this book give metric and imperial measurements for liquid and dry ingredients as well as temperatures. In the US, people often use cups to measure, so the US standards are below to show how they relate; use these for converting ingredients in recipes from the US.

## LIQUID MEASUREMENTS

| Metric | Imperial | US Standard |
|---|---|---|
| 1.25 millilitres (ml) | — | ¼ teaspoon (tsp) |
| 2.5ml | — | ½ tsp |
| 5.0ml | — | 1 tsp |
| 7.5ml | — | ½ tablespoon (tbsp; 1½ tsp) |
| 15ml | ½ fluid ounce (fl oz) | 1 tbsp (3 tsp) |
| 30ml | 1fl oz | ⅛ cup (2 tbsp) |
| 60ml | 2fl oz | ¼ cup (4 tbsp) |
| 80ml | 2½fl oz | ⅓ cup (5 tbsp) |
| 120ml | 4fl oz | ½ cup (8 tbsp) |
| 160ml | 5⅓fl oz | ⅔ cup (10 tbsp) |
| 180ml | 6fl oz | ¾ cup (12 tbsp) |
| 240ml | 8fl oz (½ pint) | 1 cup (16 tbsp) |
| 480ml | 16fl oz (1 pint) | 2 cups |
| 960ml | 32fl oz (1 quart) | 4 cups |
| 4 litres | 128fl oz (1 gallon) | 4 quarts |

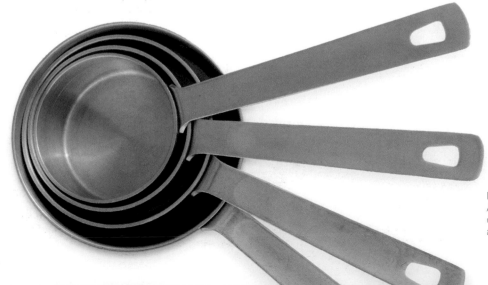

**DRY MEASURING CUPS**
A good set of measuring cups is essential for accurate cooking.

## DRY MEASURES

| Metric | US Standard |
| --- | --- |
| 30grams (g) | 1 ounce (oz) |
| 60g | 2oz |
| 115g | 4oz (¼ pound (lb)) |
| 140g | 5oz (⅓lb) |
| 175g | 6oz |
| 200g | 7oz |
| 225g | 8oz (½lb) |
| 300g | 10oz (⅔lb) |
| 350g | 12oz (¾lb) |
| 400g | 14oz |
| 425g | 15oz |
| 450g | 16oz (1lb) |
| 900g | 32oz (2lb) |

## TEMPERATURES

| Degrees Fahrenheit | Degrees Celsius |
| --- | --- |
| 110 | 225 |
| 130 | 250 |
| 140 | 275 |
| 150 | 300 |
| 160 | 325 |
| 180 | 350 |
| 190 | 375 |
| 200 | 400 |
| 220 | 425 |
| 230 | 450 |

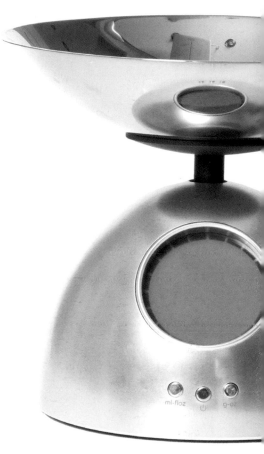

**KITCHEN SCALE**
Measuring ingredients by weight is more accurate than by volume. On the whole, liquids are given as volumes, not weights.

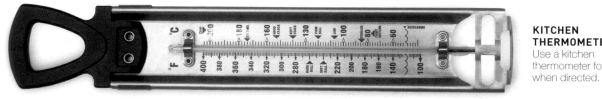

**KITCHEN THERMOMETER**
Use a kitchen thermometer for liquids when directed.

# Recipes by **Nutrient Content**

## ⊙ Fat Conscious

**Keeps calories down to avoid weight gain and promote cardiovascular health.**

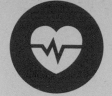

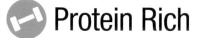

# Protein Rich

**Gives fuel for strength and rebuilding muscle.**

# Carbohydrate Rich

Provides important fuel for
endurance activities.

Apple Cinnamon Refresher, **104**

Basil Penne Pasta with Asparagus and Feta,
   **160**

Bean and Vegetable Soup, **72**

Blueberry Banana Recovery Smoothie, **132**

Blueberry Lavender Lemonade, **130**

Blueberry Madness Bars, **62**

Blueberry Orange Parfaits, **98**

Buffalo Chicken Pizza, **175**

Chicken with Orzo Pasta, **164**

Chickpea and Cauliflower Tacos, **88**

Cranberry Limeade, **50**

Creamy Orange and Carrot Smoothie, **106**

Easy Minestrone Soup, **148**

Easy Slow Cooker Pumpkin Pie Rice Pudding,
   **140**

Egg and Avocado Breakfast Burritos, **56**

Gingerade, **131**

Greek Pasta Salad, **122**

Green Monster Smoothie, **134**

Hearty Legume and Beef Soup, **144**

Kiwi Pineapple Chia Smoothie, **132**

Lavender Lemonade Relaxer, **102**

Lean, Green, Broccoli Smoothie, **106**

Lean Steak and Brown Rice Stir-Fry, **161**

Lentil Soup, **74**

Low-Fat Banana Bread, **114**

Mango Cooler, **102**

Marinated Greek Orzo Salad, **154**

Mediterranean Quinoa Salad, **150**

Mediterranean Salmon Wraps, **138**

Orange and Ginger Muffins, **70**

Peaches and Cream Smoothie, **134**

Pineapple Basil Mojito, **129**

Prawn and Spinach Pasta, **91**

Quick and Easy Energy Bars, **69**

Quick Tortellini Salad, **120**

Raisin Bran Cookies, **66**

Raspberry Lemonade, **129**

Roasted Butternut Squash, **177**

Slow Cooker Beef and Cabbage, **166**

Slow Cooker Rice Pudding, **96**

Spaghetti with Meat Sauce, **167**

Spaghetti with Turkey Pesto Meatballs, **169**

Strawberry and Yoghurt Ice Lollies, **97**

Strawberry Shortcake Milkshakes, **180**

Sweet and Salty Peanut Bars, **60**

Three Cheese and Spinach Stuffed Shells,
   **90**

Turkey Chilli, **145**

Vegetable Stew, **142**

White Beans and Broccoli, **159**

Wholemeal and Oat Pancakes, **82**

Wholemeal Turkey and Veggie Pitta
   Sandwich, **59**

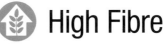

# High Fibre

Ideal for larger meals 3–5 hours
before activity.

Basil Penne Pasta with Asparagus and Feta, **160**

Bean and Vegetable Soup, **72**

Beef, Broccoli, and Sweet Potato Stir-Fry, **92**

Blueberry Orange Parfaits, **98**

Chickpea, Tomato, and Mozzarella Salad with
   Pesto, **156**

Chickpea and Cauliflower Tacos, **88**

Chickpea Salad, **77**

Easy Minestrone Soup, **148**

Egg and Avocado Breakfast Burritos, **56**

Greek Pasta Salad, **122**

Hearty Legume and Beef Soup, **144**

Kiwi Pineapple Chia Smoothie, **132**

Lean, Green, Broccoli Smoothie, **106**

Lentil Soup, **74**

Mediterranean Quinoa Salad, **150**

Quick and Easy Energy Bars, **69**

Reduced-Fat Creamed Spinach, **178**

Reduced-Fat Tuna Melts, **136**

Roasted Butternut Squash, **177**

Spicy Beef and Pasta Casserole, **125**

Sweet and Salty Peanut Bars, **60**

Three Cheese and Spinach Stuffed Shells, **90**

Turkey Chilli, **145**

Vegetable and Crab Soup, **75**

Vegetable Stew, **142**

White Beans and Broccoli, **159**

Wholemeal and Oat Pancakes, **82**

Wholemeal Turkey and Veggie Pitta Sandwich,
   **59**

# Easily Digestible

Low-fibre foods suitable for easy digestion before competition and during recovery.

# Index

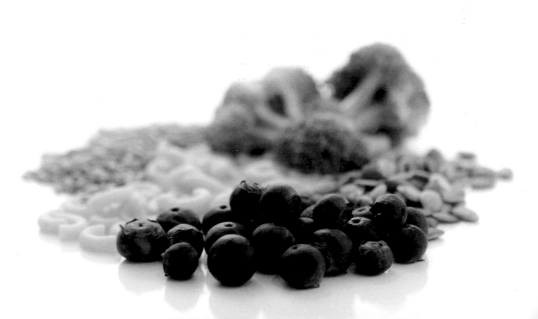

# About the **Authors**

**ROWENA VISAGIE, RD, BSc (Med) Nutrition and Dietetics,** is a registered dietitian at Shelly Meltzer & Associates based at the Sports Science Institute of South Africa in Newlands, Cape Town. She completed an honours degree in Sports Science at the University of Stellenbosch and an honours degree in Nutrition and Dietetics at UCT. She also has an IOC diploma in Sports Nutrition. Her current work in private practice includes consulting with individuals and teams of all sports and levels. She was also previously an elite triathlete competing at an international level, and more recently a social runner and mountain biker, but has put her sporting career on hold to be a mother.

**KARLIEN DUVENAGE, RD, BSc,** is a registered dietitian and head of the Gauteng Branch of Shelly Meltzer & Associates. She has extensive sports nutrition experience, having worked with both recreational and elite athletes in many sporting codes, and has also been involved in various corporate and wellness programmes. She is a popular speaker to a wide variety of groups such as athletes, coaches, and the public, and regularly writes for magazines and newspapers.

**SHELLY MELTZER, RD, MSc (Med) Nutrition and Dietetics,** is a registered dietician and head of the Dietary Practice at the Sports Science Institute of South Africa. She has close to 30 years' experience and has consulted with many national and international athletes across a spectrum of sports from recreational to Olympic level. Shelly is a part-time lecturer and research supervisor for post-graduate students in the Department of Human Biology at the University of Cape Town, and is a Faculty member of the Sri Ramachandra Arthroscopy & Sports Sciences Centre, in Chennai India. She has authored and co-authored books, chapters, and academic papers, and has developed online nutrition courses.

# Acknowledgments

Special thanks to chef and photographer Tom Hirschfeld (bonafidefarm food.com) for his exquisite photography. Many thanks also to Anthony Armstrong, executive chef at Nicolina's and director of food and beverage for the Indianapolis Wyndham West, for help in preparing the dishes for the photos. Thanks to Tara Deal Rochford, ACE Certified Personal Trainer and food blogger at Treble in the Kitchen (trebleinthe kitchen.com), for her thorough testing of each recipe. And thanks to Nigel Wright of XAB Design (xabdesign.com), for his masterful art direction and prop styling. We also would like to thank our families and friends for their constant support and encouragement.

## PICTURE CREDITS

Dorling Kindersley would like to thank the following for their kind permission to reproduce their photographs:

8–9 istock©pixitive, istock©4x6. 15 Dave King, Ian O'Leary. 16 Ian O'Leary. 11 Zygote Media Group. 12 William Reavell. 13 Zygote Media Group. 20–21 Ian O'Leary. 25 Dave King. 34 Dave King, Peter Anderson, William Reavell, Roger Norum, Howard Shooter. 35 Steve Gorton, Julio Rochon, 38 Dave King. 39 Philip Wilkins. 48-49 istock©pixitive, istock©4x6. 100-101 istock©pixitive, istock©4x6. 126–127 istock©pixitive, istock©4x6. 185 Dave King, Clive Bozzard-Hill.

All other images Tom Hirschfeld.